Introducti

'The strongest, bravest thing we can

~

Cheryl Strayed

As I settle into that precious window of time so fastidiously reserved, a strange paralysis sweeps over me. I sit poised yet immobile on my little turquoise sofa that I've set up with a tiny foldaway desk at one end of my bedroom. It's my writing corner. Well, actually it's more of a thinking corner at the moment. From here, I can make out the tips of pine covered hills that majestically border my adopted new city to the East. The contrast of emerald green against the cloudless azure sky tempts me. I've spent the day thus far alternating between daydreams of sunny hikes with my dog and the numb panic of minutes ticking by whilst not a thing is achieved.

Staring gormlessly at the screen, mind and fingers frozen, in some kind of creative stupor, is frustrating. This isn't unusual. Many writers, so I'm told, have mental blockages at some stage or another. Although, I can hardly claim to be a 'writer'. I do write poetry, prose, odd little paragraphs and ideas that come to mind, and of course lists – I have a whole book of those – but I'm not a writer. Yet. And at this rate, never will be! This is my fear. Having started this book over six years ago, I sometimes wonder if I'm ever going to finish. We have a rather symbiotic love/hate relationship. I can be passionately drawn to getting it done and at others, I don't even want to look at it. But then given my chosen subject, it's hardly surprising.

1

Why would anyone who has tried to leave behind a life fraught with heartache, as soon as the going gets better, willingly trawl through all the grit and grime they left behind? Why would they choose to revisit parts of a life that for so long they wished to jettison? I should be focusing my attentions on this new, exciting adventure in Spain.

I've always wanted to live here. A childhood dream that's become reality. But here I am, raking over old coals. Maybe it's therapy. I am a great believer in self-help, so yes, it's a little bit that. But it's also more. It's the desire to turn all the horrible crap into something good. It's the rebellious me having the last laugh at infertility's expense. It's the resilient me conquering the climb and planting a humungous great flapping flag at the top of it. 'Screw you, infertility. You didn't beat me! I'm standing strong and proud. Hurrah!'

Infertility has been my constant companion for almost 10 years. Mean and corrosive, it's been an unwelcome interloper in my marriage. It has lurked in the shadows and stalked me in the open. It's been my nemesis. It is millions of women's and men's nemesis. Since starting my research, I've been taken aback at how many of us there are. The more open I've been about my own struggles, the more I've encountered fascinating, moving and courageous stories of other inspirational people. Some were strangers who I never saw again who, in a chance encounter at a wedding, in a beauty salon, on a plane, shared their pain very candidly.

This is another reason I feel compelled to write about it, to create an insightful book that shines light into the murky, still widely misunderstood, depths of infertility. I want to talk about it, to lift the lid and expose infertility for what it really is. I do question if my husband and I really want to expose our lives in this way. But I always arrive at the same conclusion; that if it helps at least one other couple, or educates a handful of uninformed folk, then, yes, it'll be worth it.

People should know the truth. By sharing my story, I pay tribute to other infertility sufferers and what they've been through too. And for those who are still quietly year on year, battling through and getting on with it despite the burdens they carry, the strong desire to be a mother yet knowing that it's possibly a futile cause. I feel a compulsion to write it for them also. If this is you, if my story reflects part of yours, I hope this book helps you go forth with courage, strength and renewed optimism. To all those struggling to overcome infertility, this book is for you.

So, my mission and motivation are clear, yet I feel overwhelmed by the task ahead. But I must finish. At the very least, for my own well-being, and not to disappoint those who've encouraged me; applauding my poetry, reminding me to tell the truth, and spurring me on.

Now, as each face, and encouragement crystallises in my mind's eye, the words a good friend has often said to me also come into focus, 'You can totally do this!' Slowly, my hovering, immobile fingers tentatively start to type.

Procrastination

m0nnZ9kPQI

I'll cook a lasagne in a minute,
then I'll go for a jog.
Perhaps a bit of exercise
will help clear my cerebral fog.

I've been sitting here all morning
waiting for inspiration to strike,
but so far amongst what I've produced,
there's nothing much to like.

Maybe I'm just not good enough.
Maybe I'm not made for such sedentary grind.
Every few minutes thoughts of giving up
flit through my treacherous mind.

I file my nails, make more tea,
dithering and delaying,
avoiding temptation from the internet,
those online games I could be playing.

Panic sets in as the hours tick by,
still I lack motivation.
Despite digging deep to find focus,
all I've unearthed is procrastination.

Other people seem far more efficient.
They're disciplined, hard-core machines.
They rattle through words in the blink of an eye
with a work ethic that borders obscene.

I want to be a woman on a mission
whose fingers make the keyboard burn,
eroding the letters on the poor little keys
due to the speed at which my genius is churned.

When I get up early at the crack of dawn,
I want to see the fruit of my labour
rather than sat unproductive for hours
with not a thing of merit on paper.

It used to be said perfectionists waste time.
If that were true then I must be really supreme.
It used to be said that it's not laziness,
but fear of not accomplishing our dreams.

I want productivity not lethargy.
I want my brain to spring into action!
I'd like to stop faffing about,
enticed by every trivial distraction!

I feel I've an important message,
something I've just got to write.
But if it is so damn important,
why does it put up such a fight?

Words should flow far more easily!
It's not like I've got nothing to say.
There's a torrent of stuff waiting to come out.
I've just got to find a way

to get this process kick started,
to cause my synapses to spark!
At this rate I'll be here 'til Christmas
sat here alone in the dark!

CHAPTER 1
Defining infertility

'Anyone that's been in the place of wanting another child or wanting a child knows the disappointment, the pain, and the loss that you go through trying and struggling with fertility.'

~

Nicole Kidman

Before we begin, I should clarify what infertility is *not*. Like many, I've encountered some surprising misconceptions. (Please excuse the pun!) Infertility is *not* a melodramatic cry for help because it's taken a couple a bit longer than usual to conceive. It is *not* a hypochondriac's attention seeking device because they can't get pregnant when everyone else is. It is also *not* a green light for others who don't know the facts, diagnosis or details to give their own full-blown assessment of the issue, and how to go about fixing it. It isn't in any way a 'pull your socks up, don't make such a fuss, we've all got problems, try not to think about it, love' type of situation. All of which are attitudes I've come across, even from intelligent, empathic people.

I didn't intend to start with a moan. That's not the intention of this book. But it needed to be said, and now we've got it out of the way, let's move on to what infertility actually *is*. The WHO's [1] clinical definition of infertility is 'a disease of the reproductive system defined by the failure to achieve a clinical pregnancy after 12 months or more of regular unprotected sexual intercourse.' The UN's 'Convention on the Rights of Persons with Disabilities' which is an international human rights treaty, ranks infertility as the 5th highest serious global disability among populations under the age of 60. A disease and a disability! Powerful terminology. Yet even though we live in an age of deconstructing social taboos, with easy access to almost limitless information, infertility often remains an overlooked, underestimated and frequently misunderstood condition that more often than not, requires treatment.

For the 1 in 6 couples in the UK who experience difficulties conceiving, infertility is a delicate, draining, emotional, often expensive predicament. As anyone who has experienced years of unresolved infertility will tell you, it's a real pain in the derrière - quite literally if you go down the injecting bonanza that is the IVF route! Which explains why the women who have spoken to me about their own exhausting journeys feel so passionately about this topic. Many talked about feeling alone, alienated from peer groups, work environments, and families.

In the early days of my own struggle, few places offered sanctuary from the perpetual feed of procreation, pregnancy, and proud parents. Accosted by our child-centric society, I felt trapped and alone, like I was the only one in my small corner of the globe scrabbling to keep all my marbles in place, and as if no one really understood what I was going through. And yet some do.

Although difficult to ascertain an exact figure, studies show that at least 50 million couples worldwide experience infertility in one form or another,[2] affecting up to 15% of reproductive-aged couples. Global fertility rates have almost halved in the last 50 years. Obviously, there are many contributing factors, reproductive issues, disease, poor diet, environmental issues, lifestyle, stress, not enough sex... Actually, most reports don't officially give the latter as a significant factor, (some do!) but it should probably rank quite highly on the list. In the UK, in our increasingly busy, stressed, exhausting, distracted and time pressured postmodern lives, it's a wonder that anyone manages to conceive at all!

Finding the energy and compulsion to have regular intercourse with one's partner can be problematic in itself!

My husband and I were asked on numerous occasions without a hint of irony, if we were having enough sex to get pregnant? (Asked by doctors, I should hasten to add! Oh, now I think of it, and some oddly inappropriate folk who felt compelled to hand out their own special blend of sex life advice!) Defending one's intimate love making experiences, or rather 'let's bonk quickly before we pass out from exhaustion' antics to complete strangers before they begin to take your problem seriously, felt too personal and unnecessary back then. (Little did I know what lay in store, and how liberal I'd become with gory details of our bodily functions.) Checking a patient's sex life must be a valid line of enquiry, otherwise they wouldn't bother to ask.

Years of infertility is bleak and depressing. It is also weirdly absurd. By absurd, I mean funny. Darkly so. My husband and I have faced such bizarrely comic moments that at times, it felt like being in our version of The Truman Show. Or like living on the set of Beadle's About expecting the late Jeremy Beadle himself to jump out from behind a potted plant, whip off a cunning disguise, to reveal that we're the butt of an elaborate hoax! (These 'is this really happening' moments are the inspiration behind many of the poems.)

Infertility is a smorgasbord of bonkers experiences that a regular, non-fertility challenged person, would never have to face. Naturally, it's difficult, nigh on impossible, to fully comprehend it unless you've been through something like this yourself. Hence the reason why I feel compelled to raise awareness. I feel passionately that were there greater understanding of the wider ramifications of infertility, the more compassion and help there would be for sufferers.

Evidence shows that couples going through infertility cope better when they've a robust network of support and understanding around them. Understanding breeds empathy. And we *all* need empathic people in our lives, not just those going through tough times. If positive conversations are sparked as a result of reading a particular chapter or poem, then my attempt to contribute to better support for individuals from partners, friends, families, colleagues, and employers will have been successful.

During my toughest, most rock bottom moments when overwhelmed by IVF failure and trying to be an all-singing, all-dancing stepmother, wife, friend, teacher and colleague, I felt unable to openly discuss how much I was struggling. I felt ashamed. I felt I was a failure. Had I more opportunities to talk to others experiencing similar problems, it would've certainly helped. I read books, articles and very helpful forums, but in the early days I had few insightful, encouraging conversations with those who really understood.

Oh, I read recipe books too, trying out recipe after fertility boosting recipe! (I've still got a library's worth full of these should anyone be interested.) But what I actually could've done with was more advice on what to expect and how to cope with the emotional and practical elements of infertility. I also could've done with laughing a lot more! So, I sincerely hope that one or two of my poems make you laugh, or smile, perhaps shed a bottled up tear, and remind you that you're not alone.

Pure Delusion

D0HI75zqDV

Still no sign of a baby.
Still all barren and bare.
No bun in the oven.
No anything, anywhere.

Still empty and waiting.
Still counting the days.
Endless, frustrating
baby shower parties.

Still pretending not to notice
a million mothers walk past.
Suppressing the ache
with a terrible, fake laugh.

Vitamins, potions,
tablets galore.
Bonking my husband
like a desperate whore.

Another month gone,
still full of grief
for the life that I want,
but cannot conceive.

Losing my faith
and along with it hope
that it'll ever happen.
It's a really sick joke.

A test of a marriage.
For better, for worse.
We never expected
the infertility curse.

The worry of age.
My biological clock.
Terrible thoughts of using
another man's cock!

Losing my grip
on these whirling emotions.
Crying in Waitrose.
Causing commotions.

My femininity in question.
A redundant, duff womb!
An incomplete woman!
An imposter, a loon!

Ignoring friend's babies
for fear that I'll crack.
If I held one a moment,
I may not give it back!

Flippant remarks,
unhelpful words.
Just no idea
of this ongoing hurt.

'Don't think about it',
said so ignorantly.
Years of my life
thrown right back at me.

A change of direction,
that's what's required
to boost my morale,
be re-engaged, re-inspired.

An action-packed life,
managing things well.
Counting my blessings
when friends speak of hell.

Of persistent insomnia.
Nights without sleep.
While for me, it's a bonus,
a blessed relief.

I can lie in till 10,
or siesta at two
with no threat of tantrums,
drool, sick or poo!

I look on the bright side.
Am thankful for a lot.
I learn not to forget to
'To be grateful for what I've got!'.

Then all of a sudden,
my chest starts to ache.
Another announcement.
That's all it takes.

Again all alone.
Trapped in this cycle
of endurance and fatigue,
physical and mental.

I want to hear 'Mummy'.
A new baby's cry.
To have my child with me,
not a week then, 'Goodbye'.

I want to know motherhood.
Present a child to my mum.
A way to say thank you
for the friend she's become.

Phone calls at midnight.
A calm, listening ear.
Plenty of hugs
soothing my fear.

Back to prodding and poking,
appointments and queues.
Undignified positions.
More time in loos!

More peeing on sticks,
far Eastern cures.
More consultants and nurses.
What more to endure?

The worry, the stress,
the fear and confusion.
Having a baby?
It's just pure delusion!

CHAPTER 2
Nature or nurture

'Of all the rights of women, the greatest is to be a mother.'

~

Lin Yutang

For some women and indeed men, becoming a parent is life's calling, their raison d'être. They want children, feeling strongly about it from a young age. Years ago, more than one friend told me that they loved babies so much, their life goal was to be a mother to multiple children. Motherhood, above all else, was their ultimate ambition. Not unusual.

In my early twenties, another good friend told me she fantasised about babies. When out grocery shopping in the supermarket, she'd wander off-piste browsing rails of tiny baby-grows in the children's clothing section. Even purchasing items for when they might be of use. In my late twenties and single, another friend, shared that she often contemplated name combinations of future offspring, what they might look like, and motherhood.

Although, I recall questioning the sanity of my stockpiling friend, I soon learnt these are normal thoughts. Wanting children is a valid, understandable desire. Not only are we biologically predetermined to have to consider and be responsible for our fertility on a monthly basis, an element of social conditioning is attached to parenthood too. As a society we're increasingly bombarded and indisputably influenced by social trends and behaviours popularised by a media and high-profile figures who seem obsessed with pregnancy and babies. Take Beyoncé for example who raved in her 2013 TV documentary. '[It was] the most beautiful experience of my life. It was amazing. I felt like God was giving me a chance to assist in a miracle. You're playing a part in a much bigger show...' Thanks for that, Beyoncé! Very helpful!

I don't know about you, but my social media feeds are chock-a-block with advertising for mums, stories and articles about motherhood, breaking news of which royal family member or celebrity is pregnant, photos, videos and anecdotes of various offspring. I don't begrudge those who've been able to become parents. I'm not a spitting ball of furious resentment! I wouldn't wish infertility on anyone. I'm just saying that in a society where kids are treated as demi-gods, and the act of having children widely considered as one of the greatest accomplishments, we can be subliminally coerced into believing that motherhood is the pinnacle of a woman's role in society. You manage that, you've reached Platinum club status! Membership to which isn't permitted to the childless whether by choice or not.

Not all women have an urge to procreate. It fascinates me how some of us, pretty early on, before we've even left our teens, know that kids are not for us. We're marvellously complex, varied creatures! I wonder if the drive to have children, or not, is shaped more by nature or nurture. Many studies suggest that 'baby fever', the strong longing for a child, is a product of both; social construct, and our own individual biological make-up. How we are nurtured and cared for as children, our childhood experiences and relationships with our own parents, are significant determining factors in our emotional outlooks as adults. Most child development studies tell us that our early relationships with our own caregivers and past experiences greatly influence our decisions to have children, and the type of parents we ultimately become ourselves.

I grew up with an innate sense that I would be a mother. However, having children wasn't a driving force in my life. Before becoming a stepmother, and before infertility struck, the sight of a baby didn't trigger hormones that made me weak at the knees or yearn for a child. You wouldn't find me at the front of the queue at new-born debut viewings. I'm afraid I found extreme cooing and clucking over the offspring of others mildly irritating. In my twenties, to me children seemed a distant, non-priority. It's funny how things change so quickly.

As a child, I wasn't particularly 'girly'. (Not terminology, I like. What exactly *is* '*girly*'? However, it'll have to do in this instance.) I didn't have the prerequisite 80s dolls; bashed, plastic babies with blinking eyelids and unkempt hair; crumpled-faced cabbage patch kids; Tiny Tears etc. Although, I do remember a small and fairly life like doll called Paul of whom I was quite fond. A good example of that social conditioning from a young age? Already copying my mum, pretending to be a mummy myself. And then of course, when biology kicks in, your period starts and whoosh, there's that monthly reminder of what your body is naturally programmed to do.

As I grew older, I became more aware of the benefits of a strong family unit. Providing it's functional, supportive and healthy, being close to your family and having them around is great! My appreciation was due largely to the fact that my parents were... are, extraordinarily good people, and very good parents. I'm aware that not everyone is so fortunate in this regard. My brother and I enjoyed, and still do, being with them. Family provided happiness, and so was important. I felt safe, contented and loved when we were together. It made sense that I'd want to continue this with children of my own one day.

Growing up, my childhood Sunday mornings consisted of long mornings in church, surrounded by young families with ever-multiplying, hordes of children. Listening to male led and dominated sermons whilst the female congregation ran the crèche, Sunday School, and served tea, shaped my future outlook in a variety of ways. Strong visionary female role models, spokeswomen, leaders and speakers were not a priority in that environment.

Get married. Have kids. Be a wife and mother. This was the school of thought promoted by many branches of the church from what I can fathom in the UK during the 70s, 80s and 90s. It had a very particular stance regarding a woman's role. Having children was an accomplishment, and an encouraged rite of passage for a young woman. And if you didn't, you risked feeling a misfit. I was at odds with the advocacy that a woman's primary function was to procreate and be a homemaker.

Consequently, even at a young age, the representation of women felt unbalanced and un-inspirational. A square peg in a round hole, I agreed with the main principles of compassion, love and respect, but rebelled against what I felt was a hierarchical, anti-feminist, restrictive interpretation of male and female roles. My stance was that we, in equality with our male counterparts, should be actively encouraged to aspire to more than the principal duty of child-carer.

Of course, there is nothing wrong with this if that's what we want. Except, in my teens, I knew that wasn't enough. Surely, I reasoned, a woman must forge her own path to know herself more fully before she did these things? Why were so many in such a rush to leave school, get engaged, married or have babies? I longed to learn, study, explore, travel, and meet people from other communities and cultures. (My small provincial town on the Dorset coast was hardly awash with diversity.) I felt a natural pull to learn more about life and myself first. I dreamt of travel, creativity, choice, and independence.

Naturally then, after leaving school at 18, I made the most of relative freedom. After a year travelling Europe, four years at university, a year working in France, and another year of travel, it was time to pick a career. Teaching I hoped, would be a good fit for my varied and at times, eclectic skill set! This marvellous kaleidoscope of pedagogy, education, child development and human psychology has since proved to be a great match for me.

Indubitably, my attempts to educate other people's children have driven me to the outer edges of sanity countless times. Likewise, the crackers and unrealistic expectations heaped on the teaching profession's shoulders. TV programs portraying teachers as chilled out, tea-guzzling, staff room dwellers, has rarely been my version of reality.

For the first few years, I lived and breathed work, regularly putting in 60 plus hour weeks. I wasn't Bridget Jones. I had social interaction outside work, but I lived alone, often spending weekends clawing my way out from under piles of assessments, planning and books. So, as far as family planning was concerned, even if I'd had the inclination to fantasise about future progeny, I didn't have the time, nor the mental capacity to do anything about it. And as reproduction rather crucially requires a suitable male companion, procreation in my mid to late twenties wasn't remotely on the cards.

The Parent Plan

4Ue4065njo

Motherhood was my life ambition,
leave school, have a baby my only mission.
Someone to love who'll love me back,
a family of my own, no more than that.

        Seemed a good idea at the time,
        loans, degrees, parties, cheap student union wine!
        Teachers, parents, told me 'Get an education.'
        My CVs full of qualifications.

After the first, a second came along,
that's when Mr Right turned into Mr Wrong.
Out with mates, or playing computer game vids,
argued till he left, didn't want two lousy kids.

        A gap year ticket, a different monthly destination.
        Thai backpacker retreats. Indian meditation.
        Enjoying life while I was young,
        'buy now, pay later' after hedonistic fun.

Relentlessly grafting night and day,
no rest, worrying about bills I had to pay.
Toddler tantrums. Was I good mum?
Hardly recognised the worn out woman I'd become.

        Great new job, despite back-to-back deadlines.
        Working when I was sick, insisting I was fine.
        Reports, late nights, hundreds of email replies.
        Ready meals for one, dark circles under my eyes.

Juggling last minute shifts, mum always had them.
Never enough cash. Couldn't wait for when
I had more freedom for what I wanted to do,
quality me time, not just when locked in the loo!

        A promotion. In at dawn. No more morning run.
        A week in the Canaries, was the only time I saw the
        sun!
        Bought a house, a car, paid off student loan debt.
        Twenty years with that noose around my neck!

Their favourite place is the BMX track.
They're my heart, but it's a relief to get them off my back.
An evening college course. People said I'm mad,
but I want to be more than just a mum. Is that so bad?

        No wedding plus one, no work/life balance.
        Years online dating, still I haven't found romance.
        Biological clock ticking, I've been thinking lately
        that sperm donation might be the only way to have a
        baby.

Absorbed in my kids, I've lost the real me,
should've waited longer, didn't know how hard it'd be.
Responsibilities of motherhood, the multitasking grind,
guilt, anxiety, a permanently frazzled mind.

        Maybe I should've had different priorities,
        Taken advantage of younger, more active ovaries.
        Turning back the clock, would I change my plan?
        I'd like to have children, but I don't think I still can.

CHAPTER 3
Facts and stats

'While I have no intention of sounding alarmist or negative, it is true that the single most important determinant of a couple's fertility is the age of the female partner.'

~

Michael Dooley

Now, maybe this is where I went wrong. Perhaps this is where some of us who find ourselves childless not by choice made an error. In the excitement of exerting independence, revelling in freedom to choose, our biology is overlooked. Well, not overlooked exactly, just not prioritised. Some of us spend our most fertile, childbearing years focusing on everything else *but* procreating! Paradoxically, taking diligent measures to ensure that we *don't* get pregnant! Only to find that when we're finally ready and able to do something about it, biologically speaking having a baby isn't quite as simple as we were led to believe.

It never occurred to me that I'd have problems. Fertility issues weren't something that were discussed, or that I knew about when I was younger, and since then, never had cause to consider it. (Until obviously, one day I suddenly, quite brutally, did.) For an educated woman, this considerable 'information gap' seems alarming. Why wasn't I more aware of how my body functions? Why wasn't this important, relevant information, explained at school, for example?

Obviously, not as much was known about fertility then. Reproductive health and science have advanced in leaps and bounds in the last 40 years since Louise Brown, the first 'test tube' baby. But still, it would've been hugely advantageous to be less of an ignoramus about the finer workings of my reproductive organs when making key life decisions!

Indeed. I wish my secondary school educators had been more helpful in the area of fertility. Instead, I recall rather crude attempts to terrify us into avoiding sex altogether. The rationale was, I suppose, to cut teenage pregnancy rates which at the time was government policy in schools. Our Sex Education lessons, if you can call them that, involved being corralled into a dusty science lab by apathetic teachers who seemed so ancient and past it, that it was hard to believe they'd ever seen the anatomy of the opposite sex!

Once installed, we were then regaled with mind-boggling facts. Did you know that, in a single ejaculation, an army of millions of microscopic sperm are cannoned into the cervix in a race against time to fertilise the single, lonely egg? We were shown stomach churning images of STDs, a memorable video of naked people with bad hair kissing, and were forced to watch harrowing 70s footage of traumatic childbirth causing one of our comrades to pass out cold on the floor.

I remember finding the whole rigmarole of rolling a condom on to a banana performed by a visiting health worker extraordinarily bemusing and marginally uncomfortable. We then took turns to pass around an alien looking device which could be implanted into our arms for, voilà, no baby. The message was clear: if you so much as touch the opposite sex, you could be up the duff faster than you can say 'gonorrhoea!'

Would more informative Sex Ed classes have made any difference? Furnished with more reliable fertility facts, would I have made different choices? Possibly not. Youth tends to hoodwink us into feeling immortal with life stretching languidly before us. We've got time to do everything. At none of my crucial life intersections, did I feel the need to pay particular attention to my body's biological capabilities. There was also the issue of enlisting the right man. I wanted children, but I wasn't about to embark on parenthood with the first half decent chap I came across. It had to be someone special, and like I said, I had things to do first.

I think today's young women are more aware of this reproductive gamble. It's not exactly breaking news that the female reproductive system greatly favours a younger body to successfully procreate! Statistics show within her first year of trying, a healthy, fertile woman in her early twenties has an 86% chance of conceiving. Decent odds. The average woman in her early thirties has a 63% chance. Still more likely than unlikely.

By the time a woman hits her forties, the odds are reduced to 36% within the first twelve months. Meaning that less than four out of ten women will conceive naturally within that given window. Step out of that 12-month time frame, add another six months and it's slipped into single figures. Not a positive prognosis. Our eggs are the same age as us. As we age so do they. No wonder the number of young women freezing their eggs is rising! A good idea if you've got the cash. I wish I'd thought of that, knowing what I know now!

It's worth noting that male fertility does also decline with age, but clearly not as drastically, as the media is often keen to point out. Step forward quinquagenarian celebrity dads Hugh Grant, Mick Jagger, Micheal Douglas who've all had children well into their 50s. Being off the hook as far as menopause is concerned is a clear advantage in the baby-making stakes for our male counterparts! Come to mention it, I've long since wondered why *men*opause is deemed a befitting term for something so contrastingly gender specific. But, I digress!

When you spend as long as I have being confronted by these benchmark statistics, you get to know them pretty well. Having a fortieth birthday wobble is therefore completely understandable! Touted as a big deal number by most experts, forty is an age that can seem depressingly over the hill not only for natural conception purposes, but even more so for assisted reproduction.

I'd never been a birthday-phobe, but in the run up to my forties even thinking about this decade was enough to have me deep breathing into a paper bag! I'd already spent 7 years diligently bonking away in between 3 failed fertility treatments. (The fourth and final taking place shortly after my 41st birthday.) Past forty, I was more likely to win the EuroMillion jackpot than to conceive naturally or otherwise. My ovaries were shrivelling, and my poor aged eggs on their last legs. My time was running out!

Conversely though, and as if to contradict much of what I've just said, it transpires that mothers are actually getting older! As a result, in recent years there has been a sharp rise in the number of couples resorting to ASTs[3] to conceive. In the UK, in 1960, the average age to become a first-time mum was 23. By 2015, the Office of National Statistics states that this had risen to 28.6 years. There are many reasons why it doesn't happen when we're younger. Debt, ill-health, not finding a suitable partner, caring for other family members, economic hardship, freedom of choice, educational advances.

Improvement to women's rights and equal opportunities, particularly with regard to education, mean that we now have far greater choice than our grandmothers', or even mothers' generation. In the early 1960s, just 4% of school leavers went to university. Only a quarter of those,[4] a measly 1%, were women (which fits with my mother's recollection of undergraduates on her Geography and Geology degree in 1968 – of the 30 or so students on her course, only 3 were female). I'm going off on a bit of a tangent, but it's worth highlighting what a slog it was for us to get to where we are now in terms of equal opportunities in education.

Did you know that Cambridge was the last university in the UK to allow women to become full members and take degrees? Right up until 1948, women had been able to study there, but had been awarded diplomas rather than the full Degree of Bachelor of Arts equal to male graduates. And even then most male students weren't happy about it! *'When the question was first posited in 1897 of whether women attending Girton and Newnham should be granted Cambridge degrees equal in value to those awarded to men, male undergraduates protested by burning effigies of female scholars and throwing fireworks into the windows of women's colleges.'* [5]

Charming! What gents! Thankfully, the trend for burning images of female students, and assaulting them for their sheer audacity to expect equality has now passed, and the figures reversed. In 1962, educational attainment for women turned a real corner when funding changed, and the number of women in higher education started to increase. Fantastic! Fast forward to the early 2000s when women in postgraduate education began to outnumber men. Nowadays, it's taken as given that all school leavers in the western world, regardless of gender, can choose further education, and a career if they should so desire. More access to education, a change in attitudes, more effective birth control, more freedom of choice.

Thank goodness that the cultural expectation is no longer that a woman should be confined to the family home, working her way through a list of daily drudgery, surrounded by an army of children, ready to put supper on the table as soon as her husband walks through the door. Although, she is still perfectly entitled to if she so wishes, and if that's what floats her boat!

Hang on. I've paused as I've written this, thinking of several of my super-mum friends who do both – juggling demanding careers with busy family lives. Work all day. Come home. Taxi kids to various after school activities. Get dinner, help with homework, make packed lunches, do the washing, ironing, tidying, before finally flopping exhausted on to the sofa to listen to and counsel their husbands as they describe their busy day. Women's emancipation? Hmm... Certainly, anecdotally amongst my peers, an imbalance remains. There is work to be done to redress this balance and shift lingering gender stereotypes when it comes to expectations of a woman's role in the home. This is another book-worthy topic entirely!

I'm not man bashing. Not at all. Men, on the whole, are great! My husband is a whizz at domestic chores. Most fittingly and of his own volition, he is at this very moment merrily giving the house a once over with the vacuum cleaner!

General roles have definitely evened out. And as such, studies show that the more highly educated a woman, the more likely she is to choose to have children later on in her 30s or 40s. It's obvious, and hooray! Why shouldn't we if we want both? Except there's a catch. The later we leave it, the less fertile we are, and the more likely we are to encounter problems. The evidence is clear. A delay in trying to conceive for whatever noble, good or not so good reason carries an element of risk.

How do you have your sex?

KE4KN2IA1a

Excuse me, can I ask you,
how you have your sex?
It's just, I don't think we're doing it right.
It's making me feel quite vexed.

I'd like to conduct a survey
to uncover your toppest tips,
to find out if we're using them right,
you know, all our jiggly bits!

Although I paid attention
to Biology in back in school,
I must've forgotten, or remembered it wrong,
'cos it hasn't helped at all!

I should study to become a 'sexpert',
then perhaps it won't be such a struggle
to pop another human out
without getting in such a muddle.

Everyone else seems to manage it.
It's not a silly saga for the rest.
What have we been doing wrong?
We've been trying our very best.

Maybe it's about the angles
or perhaps the temperature?
Should we perform a special ritual
before each conjugal adventure?

We do use the correct biological bits.
I've double checked, so I am sure.
And from the umpteen books I've read,
we've no more options to explore.

So, this is why I need your help,
to solve this peculiar mystery.
Include your diagrams on the form,
then hand them in to me.

CHAPTER 4
My husband's daughter

'Mothers who give birth and mothers who adopt should both be considered "biological mothers", based on the changes that happen in their bodies when they become parents.'

~

Sarah Blaffer Hrdy

Any teacher will tell you that presiding over other people's offspring all week can be a marvellous contraceptive, particularly on Friday afternoons! Waving off the last of one's students from a packed class of noisy, tired, sweaty teenagers who only moments before had been clamouring for your attention, or whom you'd been trying to galvanise out of an afternoon stupor to finish off work before the final bell, is fantastically, soul-cheeringly liberating!

The realisation that a whole rejuvenating 48 hours without children stretched out enticingly before you was sheer relief. A feeling which magnified into an exhausted semi-hysterical delirium on the last day of term. My weekends and free-time were cherished recuperation time away from the classroom and children. So, my decision to become a stepmother came as a surprise even to me.

My husband and I became a serious item shortly before I turned 30. His daughter was a year old when we got together. Having established, after the first six months of spending time with him alone, that he was most likely the man I would marry, the three of us began spending time together. Quite quickly, a close bond grew between me and his daughter. I was taken aback by how speedily and deeply attached to her I became. I hadn't expected it.

Initially, I hadn't wanted to be involved with him, a single dad with such a young child and complex childcare arrangements. When I had realised I had feelings for him as my friend, I went to great lengths to avoid any involvement either romantic or platonic. (Which reminds me, is one automatically unsubscribed from dating websites after a certain period of inactivity? Or do you have to close the account yourself? I should probably check that my face and bio aren't still doing the rounds in cyberspace! I'll make a note to found out!)

One of my reasons for moving house, job and even county was to circumnavigate any relationship and even contact with him. Nevertheless, despite my reservations and move 100 miles away back to my home town, I couldn't shake the notion that we were meant to be together. (It may sound soppy, but I have come to believe in soul mates of sorts.) It was me who contacted him out-of-the-blue, inviting him down to the South Coast for the day.

This decision was borne of much soul-searching and months of internal dialogue. Even before our first date I'd already made important decisions, pledging to myself that if I was going to be in a relationship with him, then I would support him and build a positive relationship with his child.

It was a conscious, carefully considered manifesto. Years mentoring young students with warring parents, stepparents and friction at home had taught me if nothing else, the importance of trying to forge positive relationships between all care-givers and off-spring as far as possible. A child's mental health and well-being is hugely impacted by their relationships with all care-givers. But I knew this wouldn't be easy. I was right, it wasn't.

A conversation I had over 13 years ago with an 11-year old student I mentored springs to mind. The child's mother had a new partner and was unable to interact cordially with the father. My student told me that her mother barely spoke to her father and when she did it was brief, abrupt and they sometimes argued heatedly. She told me how sad and tense it made her to hear her mother speaking derogatorily about her father when he wasn't there. It was causing friction at home, especially as the student felt her new 'stepdad' was trying to usurp her father's role and push him out of the equation.

Then her mother became pregnant. More change. Initially, excited about her new sister, she quickly became resentful. Conflicted. She loved her sister, but the baby took up her mother's time and attention. Attention that used to be reserved solely for her. This student was feeling side-lined and neglected. Finding her place within this new familial configuration was difficult. Unsurprisingly, these pent-up feelings were affecting her work, behaviour and relationships at school, and was causing anxiety. Thankfully, for this student, the school's support department was responsive and excellent at guiding and helping her through this time. Happily, she left school a well-rounded and positive young woman.

Assisting young people with this type of scenario isn't unusual for teachers. We are among the first 'responders' when it comes to spotting mental health issues in our students often triggered by challengingly complex home lives. But this is a whole other matter, again deserving of its own book.

So, all of this to say that I was acutely aware of some of the challenges that face young people in blended families. And that might face us. I sincerely wished to minimise or avoid many of these 'anxiety triggers' in our future family.

It's usually tough for those of us starting out on our stepparenting journey. There's always a lot to consider and manage with tact, and tremendous care and awareness. Far more than for birth parents. Nothing can prepare us for the onslaught of challenges that we will face. So much is out of our control. But no matter how difficult things become, I encourage all stepparents to avoid out and out conflict.

Instead, to find ways to keep things positive even when it feels unfair or impossible, always putting the mental welfare of the child, our own mental health and the health of our relationship at the heart of our decisions whilst, and this is super hard at times, simultaneously acting with respect and kindness toward the other parents whether we see eye to eye or not. Sound tricky? It is. All we can ever do is our best, and be kind.

My approach was and still is, to co-parent my husband's daughter with care, and encourage my husband even when things were personally difficult, complicated or didn't go to plan. I didn't compete with, or attempt to take the place of, my stepdaughter's biological mother. There was more than enough room in her life for two mothers to raise and nurture her. Giving her a safe and loving second home was essential for her to be as balanced, confident, healthy and happy as possible. I didn't always get it right, but this was my rationale at the very least. *'Children develop best in secure social environments, and security includes turning to lots of different people and knowing they are there for you.'*[6]

A year into our relationship and my husband and I (we now lived together in Dorset) were regularly commuting to London and back to spend time with his daughter. Things had swiftly progressed. Swings and seesaws replaced weekends of assessments and exercise books. My free-time now consisted of adventure playgrounds, piloting a buggy through the damp streets of London, and dining in child friendly restaurants where I'd cut up food into tiny bite-sized morsels.

Together, we sought sunny spots for picnics and play, or sheltered from bucketing rain in warm, dry places for cuddles and stories. Dates with my husband didn't consist solely of this type of excursion, we made efforts to have time for just the two of us as well. But it was a far cry from what my younger self had envisaged for my future relationship and free-time!

I won't sugar-coat it. It could be nerve-wracking and stressful. My husband's daughter was so young and his relationship with her mother wasn't straight forward. Trying to get the right balance for us all was a challenge. In the months before we married, there were many times when I nearly gave up. But by then I was clearly head over heels with them both.

Establishing our relationship was not easy for my husband either, both of us felt emotionally tested so many times for different reasons, *'There was certainly an element of stirring things up emotionally speaking, a shifting of tectonic plates when we first started our relationship. I felt a responsibility to them both, separately and together; two worlds coming together, trying to combine them successfully without letting either person down or compromising my time with either of them. I felt responsibility to my daughter's mother too. I was aware that healthy, helpful, understanding relationships between all of us needed to be set up. I did try my best to do that for all of us. I knew that being a stepmum wouldn't be straight forward for my wife due to the complexities we faced.'* Bless him! He was, is, a very conscientious individual. He always tries his best, even when out of his comfort zone, especially emotions wise.

Stepparenting isn't for the faint hearted! If you know a stepparent well, no matter how 'together and positive' they outwardly seem, be sure to give them a whopper of a hug next time you see them. (At the time of editing we're in the middle of a pandemic. So perhaps it might still have to be a socially distanced hi-five, wave or holler! In any case, let them know that they're appreciated!) Like me, they may not often have much opportunity to discuss the highs and lows of their family dynamic, so any encouragement could be much appreciated.

Mentally and emotionally, those first few years were tricky. After each portion of time together, my urge to care for and nurture a child grew stronger. Exacerbated by the fact that life with and without her was so contrasting, I missed her. Hormones didn't help. Previously dormant, her visits sent them into overdrive. It wasn't unwelcome, but not having previously had such powerful urges to have a child, I was unprepared for this sudden tsunami of oxytocin! Privately, I began to struggle psychologically with her constant coming and going in our lives.

Reading up on it years later, I had a better understanding of these responses. Obviously, I missed her because I loved her. But there's more to it than that. Our bodies have physiological responses to those whom we love deeply. Meaning that when we deeply love our 'adopted' children, our emotions sooner or later, whether we want them to or not, will cause a physiological reaction.

Studies show that this is a normal, natural process helping us to become more effective additional carers. Both birth mothers and non-birth mothers, undergo neuroendocrinological changes. Mothers who haven't given birth to their offspring experience similar changes to those who have. When we become involved in the upbringing of our inherited offspring, developing deep, meaningful bonds, not only do we start producing more hormones, the structure of our brains change too. You could say that we evolve! Is it any wonder that my stepdaughter's absences at a time when I'd started to want children of my own, had such an impact?

Play parks and dirty nappies

RbSo1LEOej

Cake crumbs crunching under foot
Sticky tables, fetid air
Multi-sensory overload
Coats piled high on empty chairs

Eye-wateringly bright climbing walls
Alive with wriggling tots
Coughing, spluttering everywhere
Noses oozing germy snot

Laughter from the ball pit
From a slide an angry grizzle
Arguments on the trampoline
Refuge from freezing drizzle

Screeching, manic children
High on a sugar rush
Scrambling up knotted cargo nets
Refusing to finish lunch

Harassed Filipino nannies
Rocking wailing buggies
Eyes glued to pinging mobile phones
Atmosphere thick and muggy

Lone fathers hunched over laptops
Frowning at their screens
Cups of coffee growing cold
Oblivious to whoops and screams

Stagnant baby changing units
Dirty nappies, beakers, scattered toys
High-chairs smeared with sinister gloop
Backdrop to cacophonous noise

Hermetically sealed windowless box
Without sky or view to contemplate
Endless damp of February
Summer's freedom a drawn out wait

Dark, gloomy, dusty corners
no secret sun dappled glades
Neon plastic instead of pastel flowers
Hostage in a world of shade

Squashed entrails of beige comestibles
An inmate counting every minute
Watching fed up teenage café staff
Selling squash with additives in it

Sudden cheerful hollers
A fast-approaching joyful grin
The Champion of Hide and Seek
collects a cuddle for her win

Duty bound incarceration
sweetened by sweaty soft hugs
Sipping not-so-bad hot chocolate
From chipped lipstick-stained mugs

Gleeful eyes, flushed exhilaration
Begging for one more race
Dashing over grubby crash mats
Eager, happy smile in place

Armpit aromas, tearful whines
the setting for our family day
Slightly panic attack claustrophobic
but charming in a crowded, overpriced way

My turn to try to catch her,
arms wide ready to scoop her up
Wobbly bridge, giant slide
dangling from monkey bars out of puff

Exhausted, hot little body
carried out to the car
Another exhilarated total wipe out
at the indoor soft play park

CHAPTER 5
Trying to conceive

'It turned out to be tougher to get pregnant than I thought it would be. I tried for a long time, and it just didn't happen, to the point where getting pregnant became the greatest wish – and the greatest challenge – of my life.'

~

Helen Hunt

For any couple undergoing periods of intense pressure, I'd strongly recommend plenty of down-time together. For a relationship to work positively and effectively, this is essential. In my experience, a relationship cannot exist and strengthen without this. My husband and I did not always hit the mark as far as this was concerned but, when finances allowed, my husband made great efforts to soften the blow each time we took his daughter back to her London home. He would find a hotel deal and book the two of us in for dinner, bed and breakfast on the way back. This was our therapy. Dinner together, TV in bed, for me maybe a little cry, sleep, then a cooked breakfast in the morning followed by, if the hotel had a pool, a swim and sauna. What a treat! And sanity saving bliss.

This was our down-time. It certainly beat going straight home in the dark to our empty, childless home. This little ritual was critical to the well-being of our relationship. Our treat to re-centre ourselves and build in quality time together that thankfully we had the economic resources to look forward to occasionally and enjoy rather than what would've otherwise been a sad and joyless homecoming.

We haven't always remembered to nurture each other through the most difficult patches. There have been 'seasons' when we've overlooked and neglected to take care of our relationship and each other. Ending up, as you can imagine, having some serious consequences down the line. But as the adage goes, 'we learn from our mistakes'. One of my favourites on my long list of life mantras!

We can't always get it right. Especially when mentally speaking we're keeping rather a lot of balls in the air simultaneously. Superhuman abilities would be required for one of them not to drop sooner or later. But wisdom lies in pausing and reflecting on what went wrong and making adjustments for more balance going forward.

For me, psychologically, emotionally and even physically (due to the travelling that regularly filled our weekends) stepparenting a young child whilst struggling to have a child of my own was a lot to contend with. It has been the hardest thing I've ever had to manage, and that includes trying to teach Year 9 French on a rainy afternoon!

Before getting engaged, we agreed that having children together was important to us. As a co-parent and integral part of my stepdaughter's life, I was clear about my desire for children of my own. Being upfront and honest, we knew we were on the same page, procreationally speaking! Having a baby, was a priority when it felt right. In the meantime, promotions demanded our attention, plus we wanted to get married and buy a home together first. Our plan now seems a little contrived, scheduling pregnancy into our calendars at our own convenience as if it were that easy. But I guess that's what people do, and for them, it works.

During our first year of marriage, stability and routine was 'le mot du jour' for the three of us. As my husband had joined me in Dorset, the coast, the sea, the beach, the forest - my childhood places of comfort and sanctuary, were now on our doorstep. I hoped to share it with my husband, stepdaughter and future children. Much of our time was spent zooming up and down motorways to visit, collect or return my stepdaughter whose fluidity in our lives we continued to find emotionally difficult. By the second year of marriage, I was in a semi-permanent state of pangs, twinges and yearning to have a baby. I loved my stepdaughter. She was the epicentre of our lives. I didn't want to replace her, but it was time for a child of my own.

When first trying to conceive, most books and experts tell you get to know your cycle, have lots of sex in the middle, and let nature take its course. As the end of each month drew near, I'd be giddy at the possibility of pregnancy. A little thrill of monthly anticipation. Would this be it? A brother or sister for my stepdaughter. A grandchild for my parents. A child that didn't appear then disappear. Friends and family were announcing babies with increasing regularity. Soon it would be our turn. As the months ticked by and no pregnancy materialised, we weren't unduly perplexed. It wasn't unusual for it to take longer for some. We tried different strategies.

Articles, blogs, forums, such a marvellous wealth of information is available online. One can learn a lot. Being anonymous gives some folk a sense of security to share highly personal, intimate details with strangers. (Little did I know what lay in wait for us. Or how blasé I too would soon be when it came to describing bodily functions!) Some posts and responses were extraordinarily gruesome. What I hadn't learnt at school, the internet certainly filled in the gaps. The online fertility community has a remarkable footprint, and is hugely helpful and supportive, (particularly so when going through my first couple of IVFs.).

Meanwhile, sex became less fun and more perfunctory. I tracked and monitored my cycle, recording it in a notebook. I wasn't obsessed, just diligent. A good friend, whose first pregnancy hadn't happened immediately, reminded me that stress and tiredness can hinder conception. My growing frustrations were often eased by having a good old chat with her. She encouraged me, reminding me of her own short delay. I endeavoured to relax more. She gave me a rose quartz crystal to boost my fertility, suggesting I slept with it under my pillow. I don't think I ever did. Perhaps, I should've given it a whirl! The crystal may not have helped me conceive, but it was a reassuring symbol of her friendship during this time. I was thankful for her support as still it seemed as if everyone around me was getting pregnant with ease.

For eighteen months, my husband and I bonked away to the point of exhaustion until, with nothing to show for our efforts despite all our tweaks, tricks and faff, we admitted defeat and went to the doctor. Once through the doors of our local medical centre, still not believing anything was wrong, we explained our predicament, whereupon the inevitable tests ensued. At home we awaited the results.

The letter landed on our doormat a few weeks later. My husband opened it. He's not one who shocks easily, but scanning the document, the colour drained from his face. The strange thing was that there was no accompanying explanation, key, or obvious decoding device. Just figures, percentages and terminology decreeing 'Sperm Morphology - 1% - abnormal' which is never a word you wish to see or hear when it comes to health, particularly if a medical practitioner isn't immediately to hand.

The internet is not the place for medical diagnosis. We can convince ourselves that our leg is about to drop off when all we're experiencing is a mild bout of cramp! But in the absence of a doctor, a Google search is of course what we did. It transpired that a normal, healthy male's morphology[7] level should be between 4-14%. Therefore anyone with a measly 1% of normal sperm would certainly encounter difficulties conceiving.

No matter how many books were read, gymnastic routines were performed, early nights were had or fertility diets were followed, my husband's poor crooked little sperms would still swim about in ever decreasing circles getting nowhere fast! We were shocked. We couldn't understand it. My husband was perfectly capable of having children that much was wholly evident. What about the sperm that had become my husband's daughter? If his sperms had worked then, why weren't they working now?

Back at the medical centre, the doctor studied our results on her computer monitor. Sperm, she explained, are delicate, fragile cells and although there are 15 to 200 million of them jostling about in each millilitre of semen, only a 'few' in a normal healthy male ejaculate are ever of good enough quality to fertilise an egg. Pregnancy would either be delayed or completely prevented if there was a significant problem with the sperm. (No shit, Sherlock!) No baby had materialised because my eggs weren't being fertilised by my husband's dud sperm.

Legs akimbo

'I must use my core muscles.
Just two minutes more.'
I tell myself repeatedly whilst
upside down on our bedroom floor.
For stability, I've wedged myself
between the radiator and the door.
It's quite a challenge admittedly
and actually quite a bore.

The top of my head's now throbbing
and my muscles they now ache.
I try to cycle with more gusto,
but my arms are beginning to shake.
You must think, 'What's she up to?
Such a palaver, for goodness sake!'
But I'm desperate and this could really work.
There's an awful lot at stake.

I visualise the Olympics,
the champions whom I've seen
who've persevered and mastered
the perfect gymnastics routine.
Their mental strength is astounding.
They forge forward toward their dream.
I'm inspired, but exhausted and starkers.
Our Olympic Games are a bit obscene!

Back to the frantic cycling.
I pump my legs whilst still on my head.
My husband looks over in pity,
tucked up cosily on his side of the bed.
All he can see are my legs akimbo,
thankfully not my face that's beetroot red.
I know he thinks all this is futile.
Although that's not what he's actually said.

So I call out to him whilst puffing,
'Babe, this time it might actually work!'
I've always tried to be positive,
but it's humiliating. I feel an utter berk.
I wish we could make love spontaneously,
be free to sleep, cuddle or go berserk.
But behind the intimacy of our relationship,
the pressure of duty and functionality lurk.

All too often my fertile, ovulation window
dictates our passionate habits.
The looming shadow of obligation
means we have to get at it like rabbits.
Bleary eyed and numb with exhaustion,
stressed by work and at the end of our wits,
we summon the energy to get our jig on and
not lose faith in these fruity antics.

During the first few years, there were candles,
a little music and fairy lights.
I used to bother to shave my legs,
now they're enough to cause a fright!
I used to be the epitome of Aphrodite.
A temptress, transforming myself at night.
Now I leave my thermal socks on
to keep my feet warm and legs out of sight!

You'd certainly think that I'm crackers
if you could see my backside in the air.
Each month I'm clutching at fewer straws,
it's been years and still we haven't got anywhere.
Perhaps it is sadly pointless,
this often forced tragi-comedy affair.
But one day we might hit the jackpot,
thanks to these gymnastics extraordinaire.

CHAPTER 6
Refused treatment

'Life's not fair, is it? Some of us drink champagne in the fast lane, and some of us eat our sandwiches by the loose chippings on the A597.'

~

Victoria Wood

People's public responses to unexpected bad news differ. Some cry or get cross. Others panic. In a crisis, both my husband and I are unnervingly calm. He is a question-asker and fact-finder. I freeze. My insides tense. Assuming a blank rigid stare, I'm unflinching. This was our response to the doctor's next bit of news. No pre-amble, no subtle hint that the information might be difficult to digest, her delivery was as delicate as a juggernaut-wall collision.

In all likelihood, she'd continued, we wouldn't be able to conceive a child naturally. We would almost certainly need Assisted Reproductive Treatment, something called ICSI, a more complex variant of IVF. As I was under 40, the NHS could offer us up to three cycles of this treatment. This was her final flourish.

What? It was sudden, overwhelming and unexpected. Being told bluntly that you might not be able to conceive naturally, I think is a fundamentally difficult fact to face at first, for both partners. It's a shame that from a mental health perspective this wasn't handled in a gentler, more compassionate way. I hid it well, but I was devastated.

Our situation was made more complex as my husband's daughter had been conceived without trying. For all the drawbacks and challenges of marrying a single parent of an unplanned pregnancy, one of the great advantages, I'd erroneously assumed somewhere in my subconscious, was that when the time came, it would be pretty straight forward for us too. I never thought we'd have a problem. I'm ashamed to say, I felt cheated.

Over the following weeks, I struggled to reconcile myself with this news. It wasn't the ethics, or fear of the unknown. It was the injustice. Finding out he was going to be a father had come as a huge shock to my husband. To all intents and purposes, he'd found himself in the uncompromising position of facing parenthood with a relative stranger.

Although he has always been from the word go unflounderingly competent, reliable and supportive, I think that initially many people, myself included, were judgmental. Even as his friend when I'd found out, I'd been sceptical and critical of how he, or any man could be so irresponsible as to have put the two of them in that tricky situation. Doubting his character and integrity was another of the multitude of reasons why I'd been so at pains to avoid a relationship with him in the first place. But then all is not always as it first seems. It's easy to judge others and draw inaccurate conclusions when you don't know the full facts. I was wrong to have done so.

The scenario we now faced couldn't have been more contrasting. It wasn't supposed to be like this. The subconscious deal I'd made deep in my psyche wasn't going to plan... I'd give my all as a stepmother, and when the time came, I'd be rewarded with my own child. Work hard, be patient, wait my turn. My rationale now had a colossal spanner in the works!

Not only that, no matter how hard I tried, perplexing questions refused to leave my head. If there was such a problem, how had my stepdaughter been conceived so easily? Was she a miracle, one-off baby? If so, I wanted a miracle too. I deserved it! To date, our relationship hadn't been a bed of roses. It'd been hard-flipping-work! And now fertility treatment to boot. Why was I being punished? Give me a break!

But I don't think negatively for long. Despite first appearances our cups are rarely half empty, usually half full. And although 'unfairness' cropped up frequently, I focused on the positive. The ICSI was a light at the end of the tunnel. It could be worse. Other people have far more rubbish to deal with when it comes to health. It was hardly a life or death situation. Many couples on the planet, just like us, go through treatments to have their long-awaited baby. Sometimes needs must. You've just got to jump through a few more hoops than others to get there.

The more we understand about fertility, the more we grasp what a finely tuned enigma it is. Frankly, it's remarkable that humankind isn't yet extinct! Good grief! So many things can go wrong in the human body to prevent pregnancy, yet here we are in our masses in almost every nook and cranny of the planet. Nearly 8 billion of us roaming around. You wouldn't think infertility exists at all! But it does!

In 2014, according to the HFEA[8], 67,708 cycles of In Vitro Fertilisation were performed on 52,288 women resulting in the birth of over 15,000 babies. If my calculations are correct, over 2% of the UK population born that year are living, breathing medical miracles. In the 22 years between 1991 and 2013, there were almost a quarter of a million IVF babies born. The population of a small country. Literally, bucket loads of sperm!

Nevertheless, IVF/ICSI for us, was a new and little understood concept. None of our closest friends or family, as far as we knew, had had fertility treatment. So, on one hand, it was a relief to have a diagnosis, a solution, and a better chance to have a baby. On the other, something scary had landed in our laps.

Back at the medical centre, walking into the little room, we knew instantly that something was amiss. Our doctor greeted us with what was probably supposed to be a rueful, sympathetic smile, but was more of a condescending grimace. A distinct air of detachment wafted through the air as she handed over the IVF criteria to my husband. Her first words of doom were uttered, 'I see from your medical records that you already have a child from a previous relationship.' The rest of the conversation is difficult to recall accurately. The resounding gong of dread was clanging too loudly in my head.

The long and short of it is that if either partner already had children, NHS IVF wasn't possible regardless of why it was needed. That was part of the criteria. We weren't eligible for any fertility treatment after all. Nothing could be done. She was very sorry. Our only option, she explained, was to pay to have it privately. And that was that. This was more or less her parting statement.

In a mild state of shock again, we realised we'd just been informally dismissed and were now outstaying our welcome. We were no longer her patients. We'd been unceremoniously struck off the list. It couldn't have been more brutal if she'd launched herself across the room on her wheelie office chair, flung open the door, stuck her head into the corridor and bellowed, 'Next!'

I know our much loved, but beleaguered NHS doesn't have a bottomless pit of funding. Since 1948, it has operated in increasingly austere conditions. Tremendously underfunded, stretched to maximum capacity, short staffed and buckling under government meddling and pressure, it somehow still manages to function and serve the British public 24/7, for free. It is truly a great institution. But at that moment, what is supposed to be a comprehensive and fair system didn't seem so to me in the slightest. I couldn't understand it.

I was indignant. Whilst infertility is hardly a life-threatening condition, as a UK life-long national insurance, taxpaying citizen, I felt it was wrong to be denied treatment for a diagnosed medical issue based solely on my partner's status. It wasn't ethical. Stepparents should be supported and championed, not penalised and punished. Who was responsible for such discriminatory criteria? What about smokers receiving treatment for lung disease? Or chronic over-eaters who are fitted with gastric bands, or alcoholics with liver disease? Surely, help should be given to patients with non-self-inflicted conditions too. It wasn't fair! (1. I'm not suggesting for one moment that patients with these health issues shouldn't receive NHS assistance. Simply that I should be offered help too. 2. I am fully aware that life by its very nature isn't fair. Fairness isn't dished out according to what we think we deserve – more on this later.)

My husband, ever practical and calm, took the helm. We'd stay positive, keep perspective, start saving, come up with a plan, and book into a fertility clinic as soon as possible. But rarely is fertility that straight forward. There are many eye watering aspects to the IVF process, none more so than the cost. It's all very well blasé-ly recommending patients to go private, but it's flipping expensive! The overall price tag varies depending on the specifics of your treatment and the clinic you choose, but generally couples in the UK can expect to pay upwards of £4000.

When we first looked into it, the average cost per cycle was over £5000. Our ICSI was likely to set us back approximately £6000.

We were hardly destitute, but it was a heck of a sum to conjure up. Buying our house had wiped out our savings. And my husband's child maintenance payments, plus our loan repayments meant that we weren't flush with surplus cash. Even if we cancelled gym subscriptions, shopped at budget supermarkets, embargoed new clothes, meals out and holidays, we estimated it would take two years to raise that kind of money. Given that I'd be 34/35 by then, waiting could have a detrimental impact on a positive result. A cloud of despondency settled over us. Over me in particular.

I tried to follow people's not very helpful nor realistic advice to put it out of my mind, and focus on non-child related matters whilst we figured out what to do. But this was an impossibility. The comings and goings of my stepdaughter, by now a bubbly 6-year-old, continued to trigger waves of destabilising emotions. I cried. A lot. As soon as my head hit the pillow at night, everything would well up; frustration, helplessness, sadness, unfairness. The cruel irony of my situation became a regular nocturnal torment. Many nights I cried myself to sleep.

Hand over your cash

We can see that you're desperate,
but we cannot assist.
The computer says no,
so you're not on our list.

Yes, you've paid taxes,
in fact twenty percent
goes towards national health care.
Be assured, it's well spent.

But we're sorry to say,
that it's not spent on you.
There's not enough in the coffers
for your fertility issue.

You've not lost a limb,
you've no fatal illness.
So we simply won't fund
your health crisis.

Frankly, we've others
far more needy than you.
We know how you struggle,
but there's an outbreak of flu!

The criteria's quite clear
you have a stepchild.
So our decision's been made
and your request has been 'filed'.

If you do insist on help
you must look elsewhere.
We won't change our minds.
Our system doesn't care.

Why don't you go private?
Just hand over your cash.
They'll make you preggers
in a jiffy, a flash!

But you must understand,
that it's only a maybe.
There's no guarantee
that you will have a baby.

It's for you to decide
what to do next.
And if you cannot afford it,
then just keep having sex!

CHAPTER 7
Wicked stepmother

'The trick is to learn to have confidence in your abilities to be the best stepmum you can be, and how to be content and happy in your role.'

~

Dr Lisa Doodson

I've been asked if resentment ever got the better of me. Wanting my own child, infertility and stepmotherhood lumped together is hardly an enviable, nor compatible combination. It wouldn't be surprising if resentment had edged its way in. We are not machines. We're human, subject to a whole range of emotions whether we like it or not. An element of bitterness might've been understandable. But, hand on heart, I was never resentful of my stepdaughter despite my clashing predicament. It helped that my husband regularly thanked and supported me. I felt appreciated. Anyway, I wasn't doing it for a pat on the back. I did it because I loved them.

One of our many purposes on what often seems like a hostile and angry planet, is to love and be loved. I don't mean a sycophantic love, nor romantic love, rather a compassionate, altruistic love of humanity, meaning each other, and in fact, all of nature. So, I carried on with my co-parenting duties as best I could regardless of my own unfolding backstage farce.

In the early days, I hadn't been so assured of how my stepdaughter felt. I knew our bond was special, but it wasn't until she was about 5 years old that she labelled and articulated her feelings toward me. (Correlating more or less, with the child development perspective too.)

It was wonderful when, from her child seat in the back of the car on one of our jaunts, she unprompted piped up, 'I have four parents! Mummy, Daddy, Lorna and Aunty.' (Her mother's sister was living with them at the time.) I tell you, this unexpected joyful validation was just what I'd needed. As a stepparent it feels so damn good to have reassurance every once in a while that you're barking up the right tree and are on track with your step-offspring.

It's a complex job as there's not a one size fits all approach to stepparenting and blended families. There are multiple strategies to raising stepchildren. Parenting differs from home to home as it does from child to child even within the same family. Thereby what is right and healthy for one won't necessarily work or be beneficial for another!

I'm in awe of those who manage to co-parent with great selflessness despite their own challenging circumstances. A fantastic stepmother and childhood friend, Sarah, puts it like this, '*I naively thought that if I treated my stepson as my own and did my best for him, the rest would be easy! But it's not. They don't advertise that when you fall in love with someone who has a child.*'

Although I never thought it'd be easy per-se, I totally relate. Grafting away in the background often with little acknowledgement or thanks, often facing hostility and resentment themselves, stepparents deserve their own special day on the calendar! (There is a recognised Stepfamily Day on the 16th of September, but not a Stepmother's Day specifically.) A campaign should be started. Stepmother's and Stepfather's Day! What joy a hand-made card from nursery, complete with showering cascades of loose glitter, still sticky glue, random indecipherable shapes and big faltering felt-tip scrawl would bring to stepparents who have never been on the receiving end of such a gift despite all they do.

To me, stepmothers are the antithesis of the prevailing wicked stereotype. And yet, in our society, the very word 'stepmother' still conjures suspicion. Our public image could really do with a make-over. Selfish, unkind, and sadistic is usually how we're depicted. Take for example, Cinderella's infamously cruel and spiteful stepmother. Also, the Baroness in The Sound of Music who attempts to pack the children off to boarding school in order to separate the family. And most iconic of all, Snow White's evil stepmother who, obsessively jealous, instructs a huntsman to kill her stepdaughter and bring back her heart in a box.

What fantastic role models for us! Really great for our public persona! Interesting by the way that Walt Disney and his chums should chose such a toxic stepmother/daughter relationship to be immortalised in what was the first animated feature film.

Some of us though, it must be said, do struggle to adapt to our role. Years ago, I read an alarming online post by a recently married lady asking for advice. She wrote that when her young stepson came to stay, sometimes he would climb into her and her husband's bed for a morning cuddle. 'How lovely,' you might think, 'not every stepparent experiences such sweet and tender moments. How wonderful that she should be shown such affection.' This wasn't her attitude. Her stepson 'repulsed' her, she wrote. A birthmark on his back she found so 'revolting' that she couldn't bring herself to hug him. The boy reminded her so much of his mother that she struggled even to be near him.

I sincerely hope that family were able to get the support they needed. Rejection, even subtle and unspoken, is so easily sensed by children. Plus, single parents have a hard enough time raising a child whilst often negotiating appropriate, fair terms with an ex-partner, and managing their own grief and guilt. The last thing they need is a third party, their own spouse, causing divisions and further emotional fallout. I knew my husband whilst happy and excited about our relationship, also had concerns in that regard, *'I had mixed emotions when Lorna came into our lives. It was a change of dynamic with my daughter. Any change can be a bit worrying as a parent, you don't want it to have an adverse effect. Not that I thought it would, but there's an element of concern there obviously because you want your child to feel secure.'*

'I was concerned about how her mother might respond too. Quickly though, I felt positive. I had someone to talk to, and something happening that bought more happiness into our lives. Being with my wife took away some of the tension that I was feeling, so I felt lighter in spirit, I guess you could say. I've never felt that she was causing friction intentionally or unintentionally between my daughter and I. As a result, we both trust her one hundred percent to act with integrity with our well-being at the centre of everything. Often, I have seen that this has been to her own emotional detriment. '

Most stepmothers I've known work tirelessly behind the scenes on behalf of their stepchildren and partners. When I asked Sarah how she felt about becoming a stepmother to such a young child, she summed it up like this: a stepchild is *'part of the package'*, and it's our responsibility to ensure our partner's contact time with their child is *'positive and flows easily for both of them'*. I agree.

I think it's a surprise to some stepparents, even feeling guilty when they don't connect with, or particularly like their stepchild instantly. It can be hard, especially when children, older children in particular, struggle to accept their parent's new partner. This was not an issue I faced. My stepdaughter never had to adapt to big change in her family structure when I entered her life. This at least was fairly straight forward.

For many others though, getting the balance right and building confidence despite such obstacles takes perseverance. Just like regular parenting, good stepparenting inevitably requires a robust sense of humour and patient wisdom not to fluff it up. It requires consistency, fairness and kindness, and as the relationship develops hopefully the bond will grow too. *'Being comfortable in your role doesn't happen overnight: it takes time for everyone to get to know one another and for you to carve out your role in the family.'*[9]

Blended families and children who divide their time between two homes is increasingly common. A report on stepfamilies released by the Office of National Statistics stated that in in the UK in 2011, 11% of two parent families were stepfamilies. That's 10% of children living in a stepfamily. Of course, this figure must be much higher now. Further reports indicate that almost a third of people is now either a stepchild, step-sibling or step-parent.

Actually, the number of people fulfilling a step-parenting role is likely to be very much higher as the ONS research only focused on the families of a child's full-time residence, not including parents of secondary residences, like myself. That's a lot of people adapting to new lives and changes often with minimal support. From the social stigma angle, it seems completely incongruous that a significant level of anti-stepmother social bias should still exist.

Sometimes, when I gave my stepdaughter's young age, said how long I'd been part of her life, or when people knew I was not her 'real' mum, there could be an awkward pause, or eyebrow flicker. Even when subtle, a fleeting glance, a tone of voice or comment made me feel uncomfortable. (Now I wouldn't respond in this way, but once again that's the benefit of age, experience and wisdom.) My immediate compulsion was to want to explain our story, to justify who, why and what I was. I imagined unfair, judgmental scenarios flitting through their heads. What were people assuming? That I had lured my husband away from a young child and her mother?

Do you know, someone once more or less said this to me! It's astounding the stuff that comes out of people's mouths, but we'll get to that later. My confidence was extremely low. I could be sensitive to even a hint of criticism, but I was no fool. Thankfully, I eventually learnt how to process these judgements real and fictional, and let them go. It became easier the older my stepdaughter got too.

The emotional challenges of life with any child, birth or non-birth, is stressful sometimes. Trying to keep some semblance of balance in our lives as a trio, the 'just a stepmum' and not a 'real' mum stigma, the alienation, worry and growing shame of failing to conceive contrary to my steadily procreating peers, was all very draining. The unique set of challenges that my husband and I faced as a partnership was very different to those around us.

In retrospect, I should've capitalised on my friendship with Sarah who was also struggling to have a baby whilst trying to keep all her stepmothering plates spinning. But we were both bogged down with everything, trying not to crack up! Plus, most critically, Sarah, after years trying to conceive, was in the midst of her own trauma. Five months into her long-awaited pregnancy with her first son, it had been discovered that he had Patau Syndrome. Her son, she was told, was 'not compatible with life', and she needed to 'terminate the pregnancy'.

Dreadful. I'm in awe of how she managed to cope with the shattering grief of losing her son all the while still having to look after and care for her husband's young son. A terribly cruel twist of fate. I regret that I didn't reach out to support her as well as I might have. But I was only just managing to keep my own head above water. I wish I'd been able to offer more support. I would have a different approach now if I had my time again.

Life for new stepmothers can be as challenging as it is for new birth mothers. Some say the challenges they've faced parenting their spouses' children have been greater than those raising their own. Unfortunately, for new stepparents, when the going gets tough support isn't as readily available as it is for birth parents. When new stepfamilies are formed no one pops in to check on them. The psychological, physiological and emotional well-being of a new blended family isn't routinely monitored unless there is a flagged safeguarding issue.

When I became a stepmum it would have been helpful to have had more external support. In the UK, post-natal care for birth mothers is relatively easy to access. There are health visitors, GP referrals if required, community groups, parenting classes, NCT groups or equivalent. A fantastic range of services within the community, many free of charge, educate and assist. The parent-toddler activity groups provide a great place to meet and talk to other new parents. These didn't exist in the same way for new stepparents, especially if your spouse's child is with you for weekends and holidays only. For many stepmothers, meaningful and supportive connections with other stepparents can be difficult to find and cultivate. Little wonder that some of us, like the lady on the forum, can lose perspective and our way!

Stepmother

'Mirror, mirror on the wall,
who is the fairest of them all?'
The wicked queen demanded.
Whereupon to kill the child
the huntsman was commanded.

Into the forest the girl had fled
to escape her evil stepmother,
the woman who against all odds
was now married to her father.

We're wickedly mean, us stepmothers.
We're all cruel and calculating.
Children, I should warn you now,
our speciality is hating!

We wait till no one's looking
to exercise our spiteful greed,
then out it'll pour abundantly
to thwart you, our husband's seed.

We're too selfish to love you.
Who do you think you are, spoilt child?
We have rules, so stick to them.
Ha! Acting so innocent, meek and mild!

The household's ours to govern now.
Don't look to Daddy for explanations.
Our wicked spell has befuddled his mind,
he won't hear your whimpering protestations.

Yes. Life around here is about to change
with us now at the helm.
A new era is about to dawn,
the age of the stepmother's ruthless realm.

One last word about bitterness,
unlike the fairytale queen's fortunate quarry,
should you ever dare to cross us dear,
there'll be no happy ending to your story.

CHAPTER 8
The pre-IVF jamboree

'Money isn't the most important thing in life, but it's reasonably close to oxygen on the 'gotta have it' scale.'

~

Zig Ziglar

It may seem that rather than sticking to more fertility related matters, I've wandered off on a tangent. However, I've come to realise that in many cases stepmothering is a fertility matter. Furthermore, I'm not sure how I'd tell this story without its inclusion. Stepmotherhood was intrinsically entwined with my struggle to conceive. They were spun tight. Stepmotherhood brought me a sense of purpose and joy whilst simultaneously being my poisoned chalice. Also, it's a subject, like infertility, deserving of more public 'airtime'.

Many parallels can be drawn between some aspects of stepmotherhood and infertility. Ones that, despite living through both, weren't so apparent to me until I began to reflect and write about them. Firstly, there's the sense that although you're doing and giving your utmost as a step-parent/trying to conceive, essentially you aren't in control of your journey or destiny. You are to an extent, but many other variables over which you have limited determining say come into play. Though you have a clear idea of the direction you want to go in, the path you want to take and the outcome you'd like, it's pot luck if it works out that way. Although a cliché, 'rollercoaster' is appropriate terminology and imagery for both.

Secondly, there's the mental game. Both stepparenting and prolonged trying to conceive require mental rigour. Before embarking on both 'journeys,' I was woefully underprepared, unaware of the high levels of mental and emotional stamina that would be needed. No one told me. Just as Sarah said in the last chapter, I didn't know.

One can courageously step into the stepmothering arena having securely fastened one's Wonder Woman cape and tightened one's bootstraps, only to realise fairly quickly that a little more pre-match limbering up would have been advisable. But, by then it's too late. You're already in the ring. Trying and repeatedly failing to conceive is similar. Each month you're knocked out of the fight. You've taken a complete hammering, but you get back up again and again to face the next round until one of two things happen. You either emerge victorious, or you admit defeat and stoutly limp out of the arena to recover and review tactics for next time.

Thirdly, for both, there's the financial factor. There is a temptation to blow vast quantities of cash on a much-loved child who doesn't permanently reside in your home. With the elation of being together, the urge to overindulge beyond your capacities is strong. But as with everything in life it's a question of balance. Ensuring that your stepchild has all she needs with extra treats thrown in, yet not burning through your salary at the rate of knots due to wanting to make it special, is essential. A bit of cautious pre-planning and organisation must be applied in order to maintain economic status quo. Besides, you don't need mountains of money to make family time special, although sometimes it does more than come in handy, especially when travel and distance are involved!

If ever you were looking for a sure-fire way to deplete your bank balance, then look no further. Private IVF/ICSI is just the ticket! Multiple rounds is an investment to make even the most hardnosed high-rollers quiver. Private ICSI requires money. Fact. If you don't have several thousand, or in our case tens of thousands, of pounds, knocking about then you're out of the game.

Unfortunately, for millions of infertility sufferers around the globe finding the money is difficult. I remember once reading an article in which the journalist interviewed tribal women in sub-Saharan Africa who had given everything they had to try to have a child. Everything. Their livelihoods, their homes, borrowed money from family members to have treatment. Then when treatment was unsuccessful, they found themselves in a desperate situation. Unable to regain economic financial stability, plus labelled with the terrible social stigma of being unable to produce a child, they were rejected by their husbands, their own families, and communities for being childless. I have more to say on the social stigma of being a childless woman later.

The financial burden of repeated treatments is a strain that already stressed (and in many cases, grieving) couples could do without. My husband and I know people who got into considerable debt to fund it. Others re-mortgaged their home, sold their car, borrowed from family and even sold their house.

Our plan to save was a solid, but depressing strategy, made all the more so by the gaping hole my stepdaughter's absence caused after each visit. It was an emotional minefield for us both. But like many a good traditional tale (I'm thinking the fantastic Grimms' Brothers Fairy Tales - my favourite book as a ten-year-old) our story has a fairy godmother moment too. Step forward benevolent parents-in-law.

Being offered, not as a loan, but as a gift, the sum we needed was like being granted early release from prison. From a mental health perspective almost certainly. Nevertheless, I felt uneasy accepting their hard-earned money for potentially zero return. Incredible advances in reproductive science and all the money in the world still aren't able to guarantee a successful outcome. Statistics put us in the 36% chance of success category. It was a gamble. I desperately wanted a baby, but it seemed a frivolous expenditure when most have children for free. Obviously, there were no strings attached, it was a gift. But I feared disappointing them. Although we had ecstatically accepted, I wrangled with the notion of 'wasting' their money. So, I met with my brilliant South African colleague and friend, Karen.

This was another one of those critical points in my 'journey', when I was fortunate to have wise encouragement from someone who'd already trudged their own weary path through infertility. Having been through the IVF process four times herself, Karen's advice was insightful and timely. Accept the money, get over the guilt, they were family after all, and focus our energies, which we would need, on the treatment itself.

Her treatments had been funded by her in-laws. I was reassured. Go for it, she urged. Don't waste precious mental energy worrying about anything else. It felt good, reassuring to talk not to a doctor or medic, but to a knowledgeable friend about some of the realities of treatment before starting. Only they truly understand the impact and demands of the process.

Talking about an emotionally charged, and personal topic isn't everyone's cup of tea. Personally, it was helpful to discuss it with another like-minded woman whom I trusted. Just like when I became a stepmum, finding 'others' who understood wasn't straightforward.

Although no longer taboo, the intimate nature of infertility isn't appropriate conversational material with just anyone. Unless you've joined a local support group or online forum, discussing invasive procedures, semen analysis, sickness, injections, hormone levels, drugs, side effects and then grief isn't most people's idea of entertainment. There is such a thing as oversharing!

Once, after a failed IVF round, at a friend's glamourous Parisian wedding, I did just that – a massive overshare. Fuelled by copious amounts of champagne, having a glorious time, my husband stumbled across me gaily offloading gory IVF details to a small group of bemused guests. (To this day, I maintain that they were finding it informative and entertaining rather than repulsive!) Thankfully, he expertly intervened, gently steering me away to a quieter corner of the British Ambassador's garden! (For a Europhile such as myself, a wedding reception at the British Embassy in Paris was hugely exciting. Another reason for my headiness? Ferrero Rocher, anyone?) Anyway, my point is that it's surprising how quickly one can become desensitised to discussion of wombs, eggs and sperm, especially when sozzled!

In the grand scheme of things, £6000 seemed almost reasonable comparatively speaking. The price tags of other treatments were more. For example, if you've no useable sperm at all, you'll need to pay for donor sperm. If you do have sperm, but none in the ejaculate, like men who've a blockage or have had a vasectomy, sperm must be retrieved directly from the testis. This is extra too. When there are sperm, but no eggs or their quality is poor, you can pay to use someone else's. The charity Brilliant Beginnings estimates that surrogacy using your own eggs and sperm will set you back on average £12,000 to £15,000[10]. Almost everything is available at a price, except the guarantee that it'll work!

Surrogates are used for many reasons, repeated failure of IVF treatment, premature menopause, recurrent miscarriage, problems with the uterus... Reality star Kim Kardashian West was publicly open about their use of surrogacy for their third and fourth children. Doctors had advised her not to go through more pregnancies due to a life-threatening condition that it caused. She was honest about these surrogacies. When it's not acknowledged or talked about, it leaves the rest of us in the dark over the truth and scale of fertility related issues. So it is refreshing and reassuring when celebrities speak candidly about their fertility heartaches.

John Legend and wife, Chrissy Teigen, were insightful spokespeople about their struggle to conceive too. There are others in the media spotlight who've talked about this in recent years. Of course, the frustrating reality is that for these high profile figures the financial stress, funding limitations and economic pressures are not at all the same as it is for the majority of us. Nevertheless, shining a public light on the traumas caused by fertility problems rather than glossing over it does help raise awareness.

So, whatever your chosen route or the one you're recommended, either way it's a lot of money that doesn't always include all the hidden extra costs, for example complementary therapies or counselling. The psychological element wasn't on our radar. It was all 'positive' thinking, and the administrative, practical and physical demands of the procedure.

Now, it seems ludicrous that robust psychological preparatory care, and aftercare wasn't and still isn't, routinely included as standard practice alongside every IVF treatment. Most UK private clinic packages do offer a counselling session or two, sometimes more, with an in-house counsellor. However, not realising that this preparatory support could be very helpful, many couples don't opt for it before treatment. Why would they if they weren't made fully aware of the psychological demands? We didn't.

When I asked my sister-in-law Heidi, about her experiences during their first round of IVF, they didn't either. She had this to say, '*I could've had pre-counselling, but it was a long wait. Their psychologist only worked one day a week so got booked up quickly. I did book an appointment which ended up being the week of the transfer by which point I didn't feel I needed it. Once the IVF failed, I paid for my own counsellor. Counselling is really important. They should have more counsellors and encourage couples to talk to them as part of the preparations before starting treatment. It might have helped us more when our IVF failed.*'

Down the loo

QsUsWWP98O

Will it end up down the pan,
the best part of seven lousy grand?
It's such a waste. It's such a shame
to watch it trickle down the drain.

And if we need two or three more rounds?
That would be over twenty thousand pounds!
Let's be clear, when I say 'we'
I'm talking about the whole family.

My in-laws, parents and of course us,
will all have donated to this infertility farce.
It's a family investment, let's just say!
Raising enough just to pay

for treatment because NHS assistance
wasn't offered despite my insistence!
My husband has a daughter, he's already a dad,
so no help for me 'cos of the child he's had!

It's tough to take when you graft hard and pay tax,
help raise a child with minimal thanks.
The financial side is quite a burden,
especially when success is uncertain.

The unfairness of it, at first was depressing,
but life has since taught me to be more accepting.
For many it's worse, life really is shitty.
We've all different battles. I scored infertility.

It's shocking the amount some have paid.
For most, kids are free, you just need to get laid!
For us procreation hasn't quite gone to plan!
By now, we should have an army of babes in prams.

Let's be honest, IVF isn't a great investment.
Zero return would be a crushing disappointment!
Or thousands of pounds might get us closer
to solving this issue of no bread in my toaster!

This leads me to ponder how far we'd go,
how many treatments to implant an embryo?
Friends have sold houses, taken out huge loans,
now they have babies, but don't have their homes!

Am I cut out for a life so tight budget?
No fun weekend treats. Is it really all worth it?
A waste of resources! I'd rather it used
to send the in-laws on a Caribbean cruise.

Or buy a sports car, or luxury yacht,
skiing in winter, in summer anywhere hot.
But if it does works - relief! No more crazy spending
We will have bought a baby and our own happy ending.

CHAPTER 9
IVF – ICSI

'Per aspera ad astra.' *'Through hardship to the stars.'*

~

Latin phrase

Selecting your clinic and most suitable package is not dissimilar to finding a good Chinese restaurant and browsing set menus. Much like scrolling through restaurant reviews on TripAdvisor, clinic reviews and success rates can be found online in the UK. The HFEA has a particularly helpful website, full of advice, useful information and relatively up-to-date statistics regarding success rates which UK clinics are obliged by law to publish.

Clinic brochures and webpages explain the options with terminology and acronyms that healthy, fertile people are lucky never to have to decode and remember. Due to our abnormal sperm morphology, we'd been advised to have IVF/ICSI (Intracytoplasmic Sperm Injection) which is a technique in which a sperm cell is selected by an embryologist and injected into the egg cell. Once fertilised, the egg is cultivated for a few more days before being released into the womb where hopefully it'll implant.

When it all kicks off, there are appointments galore. Routinely juggling visits with work and family commitments demands organisation. Those unfamiliar with the process won't realise the time implications treatment entails. Our first clinic was an hour's drive away. By the time we'd finished that round, I could've driven that stretch of road blindfolded! A lot of time was spent sat obediently in rooms and corridors whose walls were adorned with sickening baby photos. Hordes of smiling new-borns held aloft by folk we recognised as staff at the clinic. Presumably the result of successful treatments.

These galleries - the waiting room décor in each of the three clinics at which we've been treated - always struck me as odd. Unnerving rather than reassuring, upsetting even, to sit hemmed in by those framed babies. What an awful place to wait once we knew our treatment hadn't worked! Mocking torture. (To make it fair, a corner of photos of crying, red eyed, blubbering couples should be provided for the unsuccessful. It might've helped us not to feel such misfits. As if we were the only ones whose miracle baby photos wouldn't be hung on those damn walls of smugness! It's important to celebrate success. But really?)

IVF is a collaboration. Consultants, nurses, and embryologists become your new buddies, everyone works towards the same goal. In the intense weeks of treatment, you see more of them than your own friends and family, discussing every aspect of your health and routine. They get to know your bodily functions better than you. I tell you, there's not much dignity when it comes to fertility treatments, particularly IVF. Scans, tests and scrutiny of one's body (sticking legs in the air in the gynaecological examination chair whilst doctors rummage around your uterus umpteen times isn't the most delightful of procedures) become your new normal. Being bashful isn't an option!

For months prior to our first IVF, at the recommendation of our consultant, I'd been seeing a fertility reflexologist to help me relax and complement treatment. (Amazing, but another hidden cost that no one tells you about until you're in the thick of it.) My husband and I tried to reduce our stress as cortisol is a recognised fertility inhibitor.

Though already quite healthy, we'd made adjustments, increasing cruciferous veg, pulses, fish etc, (but, oh, the bore of cutting down alcohol, the turgidness of lack of caffeine, the desperation of suddenly needing to pee out all that hydrating water!) What lengths one goes to in the pursuit of excellent eggs, super sperm and wonderful womb lining! Light, gentle exercise at least three times a week was also part of the fertility well-being program. Above all, we tried to spend quality time together doing nice things to feel positive and energised rather than anxious.

Then the drugs began. Boy oh boy! Wow! The drugs. There are different types of different dosage strengths. Most people are unaware of the eye-watering amount of injections involved. As if it's not already an emotional rollercoaster, you're pumped full of hormones, starting with ones that within less than two weeks (although this varies from patient to patient) supress and control your cycle, effectively switching off your ovaries - a mini-menopause. Like the real thing, side-effects include insomnia, hot flushes, mood swings, nausea, headaches and fatigue. Zombified overnight, I hit a wall! My head was gripped in a vice. Functioning at work felt like wading through mud!

Next comes the stimulation phase - synthetic hormones bring your ovaries back to life. At the same time every day, my husband administered both daily injections whilst I tried not to flinch. I'm not a needle fan and don't have much extra flesh, so by now patches on my legs that weren't already pricked, sore or bruised were scarce. A trypanophobe's nightmare! (When we'd been handed packet after packet of syringes and hypodermic needles, even we'd been bamboozled!)

Once the stimulation hormones take effect, thankfully you begin to feel less tired. But now your ovaries are growing. Rapidly. From switched off, dormant little things to juicy, ripe orange size. Meanwhile, you carry on toing and froing to the clinic for ultrasounds monitoring the ovaries' progress, for another week or two. Until finally, you get the phone call summons to the hospital for egg collection.

Egg collection is when the legendary Two Week Wait (TTW) begins. Under sedation in hospital, the eggs are removed from the ovaries by inserting a teeny tiny needle attached to a catheter into each follicle of the enlarged, stimulated ovaries to suck out the eggs. (As you can imagine piercing each ovary countless times with a needle has unpleasant side effects.)

Whilst the eggs are retrieved, the male partner is sent into a little room to produce his semen sample. (If there was ever a need to perform under pressure gents, then this is it!) Out he comes bearing his pot of gooey wrigglers that are whisked off to the lab to join the harvested eggs for fertilisation by the embryologist's magical ICSI wizardry. The eggs that do fertilise start dividing at which point they are referred to as embryos that two, three or five days later are transferred into the womb.

Oh, it's so much fun! Especially in the subsequent days as the couple wait for news. How many eggs fertilised? How many survived? What is their quality? Many UK clinics give a daily progress report. Each morning, I waited for the embryologist's call. Waiting for the first update is nerve wracking. When she phoned the morning after our transfer even she'd sounded relieved. Of my fifteen harvested eggs, eleven had fertilised. She congratulated us. I was overjoyed!

I was just as nervous, and now sore, the following day. Post-retrieval can be uncomfortable, painful for some. Empty follicles gradually fill with fluid causing the abdomen to swell alarmingly. In severe cases, bloating can be debilitating, dangerous even, leading to hospitalisation. Ovarian Hyperstimulation Syndrome, stimulating too many follicles with too high a dosage of drugs, enlarges ovaries to an uncomfortable grapefruit size. (Normally, they are roughly the size of apricots.) Patients with serious OHSS will have their eggs frozen and transfers postponed until they're well enough to continue. It's scary, painful and stressful, and happened to a friend of mine. I hadn't anticipated feeling so bruised, battered and bloated, but thankfully, my OHSS was mild.

By the third day, we'd lost two fertilised eggs. They hadn't made it through the night. The cells had stopped dividing. Though she couldn't explain why, the embryologist reassured me this was normal. Only the strongest embryos would be chosen. Everything still seemed positive. Nine, she told me, was good.

The next couple of mornings, I was anxious. Each microscopic collection of cells represented potential precious life, so it's hard not to be emotionally invested in their survival. Those nights I tried not to fret that more were fragmenting. I worried that, like another friend of mine, by the time Day 5 transfer came we'd end up with no live ones at all. But there's nothing you can do except wait. Sure enough, as the countdown to transfer ticked by, we lost more. By transfer day only five of our original 15 eggs were left. The embryologist reassured again us that this was more than enough for a successful outcome. She's right, it only takes one!

Even if every embryo survives, only a maximum of two are transferred in the same cycle in the UK. For us, and most other European countries, the legal limit is two for women under forty and no more than three over forty because, whilst multiple transfers increase the chance of success, the risk of harm to mother and foetus is also higher.

Our strict European regulations safeguard the health of patients as the first priority. The United States, however, only has recommendations. At the time of publication there was no national law governing a maximum number transferred which is how a woman can end up giving birth to triplets, quadruplets or even octuplets. As was the case in 2009, when American mother, Nadya Suleman, famously nicknamed by the media as Octomum, controversially gave birth to eight babies. In Europe, this simply couldn't happen. Every aspect of IVF is highly regulated.

Known in the trade as 'frosties', surplus embryos can be cryogenically stored for later use. Obviously, it's another additional cost. Whilst retrieving and thawing an embryo is more complex than rooting around the back of a freezer, digging out an old packet of peas and leaving them on the counter to defrost, the concept isn't dissimilar.

Although frozen embryos have a slightly lower success rate than fresh transfers, there are obvious advantages. It cuts out a part of the otherwise lengthier, costlier, more stressful process. However, not all embryos are of good enough quality for freezing. We wanted to freeze our remaining three, but sadly, they weren't deemed strong enough to survive thawing. Without this back-up option all our hopes were pinned on just two.

Holding my husband's hand, on my back, bladder full to bursting (a requirement to open the cervix as much as possible) legs splayed, staring at the ultrasound screen, we waited whilst the embryos were brought from the lab, where they'd been cultivated, to the consultant who manoeuvred the teeny syringe into the best spot for them to nestle into my velvety womb lining. Described as a quick, painless procedure, transfer was uncomfortable. I seem to possess an unusually crooked cervical canal. Yeay! Catheters, like bumper cars, dislike going around corners!

Keeping embryos alive was now my responsibility. My husband was handed an ultrasound print out of our two embryos being blasted into my womb. There wasn't much to see. We could just make out two tiny shooting stars, little dots of light, streaking across a dark, blank canvas. In hindsight, an ultrasound of embryos at this juncture seems odd. It's far from a fait accompli. You're not pregnant. You don't know if the embryos will survive. Being given a scan is psychologically misleading to a naïve and desperate couple. Isn't it better to wait for a positive result first? I had clutched the hazy image with relief, mild excitement and terrific fear. Seeing our embryos, knowing they were inside me, was the closest we'd ever knowingly come to being pregnant.

An hour later, armed with a plastic bag that rattled with pills, hormone pessaries and assorted paraphernalia, we returned home for the Two Week Wait. The TWW is a legendary. A test of mental stamina, it's normal to be driven completely loopy. What were they doing in there? Were they alive? Or had they disintegrated? Day and night willing them to survive, and implant into cushiony uterus walls.

Bursting with hormones, you swing from fierce positivity to absolute terror and back again many times daily. Each twinge and ache trigger surges of doubt or excitement. Was it a period or an implantation pain? Was I pregnant? Exhausting physically and emotionally. Those days dragged by interminably.

Waiting

6hLj8wABID

Waiting for calls, waiting for faxes
Waiting for forms, emails and taxis
Waiting for results, waiting for news
Waiting for info, answers and clues

Waiting for admin, an important letter
Waiting for consultants to tell us the matter
Waiting for side-effects that'll make me feel sick
Waiting for doctors to get it over with quick

Waiting for sleep, waiting for drugs
Waiting for an abundance of healing and hugs
Waiting for success, waiting for failure
Waiting for respite from financial mania

Waiting for blood, waiting for money
Waiting for injections to puncture my tummy
Waiting for eggs, waiting for sperm
Waiting for embryos to see if they'll form

Waiting for peace, waiting for home
Waiting for grief to leave us alone
Waiting in corridors, waiting in clinics
Waiting in hospitals, cars parks and panics

Waiting in surgeries, waiting in queues
Waiting in beds, chairs and various loos
Waiting in vain, waiting in hope
Waiting to see if our marriage'll cope

Waiting through months, waiting through years
Waiting through laughter, blood, sweat and tears
Waiting through shame, waiting through fear
Waiting to see if *that* day is finally here

Well, waiting's a joke. It's overrated
It's really quite cruel. I've grown to hate it
But, waiting's the game for the infertile few
So much time waiting, but what else can we do?

CHAPTER 10
A range of attitudes

'Words have the power to both destroy and heal. When words are
both true and kind, they can change our world.'

~

Buddha

We didn't harp on about it to every Tom, Dick and Harry! Not everyone
knew. We didn't tannoy announce it, but it wasn't a secret. It was
something we choose to be transparent about. Besides, some practical
elements obliged us to tell certain colleagues, family members and
friends. Honesty has obvious pros and cons. Telling people opens you
up to all kinds of attitudes and responses. The more others know, the
more likely you are to be at the receiving end of both helpful and not
so helpful comments.

'How exciting!' exclaimed with a beaming face, is probably the most
discordant response couples experience to the news they're embarking
on, or are mid-way through, IVF. In my poll of compatriots this came
out top as the most unsuitable remark. IVF is not a definition of
excitement! Especially for folk going through it numerous times and
who've re-mortgaged their homes to do so. Sure, there are moments
when with a tingle of excitement you dare believe it might work, but
generally the overriding sensations particularly during the Two Week
Wait, are stress, anxiety, exhaustion and fear!

'That's awesome!' is also at the top of the 'what not to say' list.
'Awesome!' would be being able to magically conceive like every other
seemingly fabulously fertile couple without months or years of

expensive stress and uncertainty. 'Awesome!' would be not reversing out of your drive into your neighbour's parked car early one morning because you're so distracted and fatigued by appointments, injections and disintegrating embryos. 'Awesome!' would be being blessed with bodies that function as they were intended rather than being subjected to undignified physical examinations, prodding and poking, feeling like an abnormal, defective human.

It's not surprising that perceptions and reality clash. That a couple may have been given a mere 25%, 12% or even less, chance of a success is often not made public. The strain that the whole palaver can put on a relationship is also, in my experience, not widely openly acknowledged. 'Exciting, fantastic and awesome' are not definitions compatible with the emotional pressure a couple is under. Many additional factors and repercussions are managed behind closed doors, so folk would be unaware of how delicate, complex and painful the Pandora's Box of infertility actually is.

Pumped full of hormones, feeling grotty and anxious, a few small words can make a real difference. There is a huge gulf between, 'IVF, that's great!' and 'IVF, that's tough. Let me know how I can help.' A contrasting emotional approach and, therefore, impact. Knowing that someone understands, or at least is prepared to try to understand if you have a wobble, is a relief!

Unintentionally glib, incongruous comments rarely come from a place of unkindness or indifference. People don't know how to help because they're unaware of what the whole procedure typically entails. That said, it surprised me how little people knew about infertility and treatment. So, although 'exciting, awesome and great' feel painfully gauche, they are often meant as encouragement.

Other humdingers consist of, 'Enjoy life whilst you don't have kids!' Or similarly, 'You're lucky you don't have any!' Some, even those we knew well, often forgot the huge part of our lives that my stepdaughter inhabited. A case of not thinking before speaking. We never held a grudge, but it did hurt to feel overlooked as a family. I asked my husband about how these comments affected him, *'Over the years, there have been a few strange comments, like 'when you have kids...' type thing. I've sensed sometimes people overlooking my role as an involved dad. Obviously, I've a lot of parenting experience, but have rarely been asked to share it, or for my advice.'*

'Sometimes, conversations about kids happen around me without acknowledging that I too, am a parent. But then, I don't chip in talking about my daughter every time, as sometimes it makes me sad depending on how long it's been since I've seen her. And I don't particularly need those sorts of emotions surfacing, getting in the way. It's nice when people do ask us about my daughter, and acknowledge that we must miss her. That we are a close-knit family unit. When there have been long periods that we've been apart both my wife and I have found that difficult. Any parent would.'

To be fair, careless words were usually uttered by people practically on their knees with exhaustion with half-scrambled minds! Young children tend to be energy-sapping, inconsiderate, complicated creatures! The benefits of life without my own were not lost on me. Increasingly, parents seem to be buckling under the strain of keeping all of their familial, personal and professional plates spinning, whilst also trying to keep their offspring alive! Little wonder I was urged, with more than a hint of wistful envy, to focus on other opportunities that I had at my seemingly unshackled childfree feet. Even so, these words aren't really appropriate for any couple struggling to have a child, least of all a stepparent.

Cue the next clanger, 'Maybe you just need to come to terms with it.' Ouch! A slap in the face would sting less. Not a phrase to be said to those who've experienced unsuccessful treatment, or indeed miscarriage. This is a galloping big no-no phrase! A dear friend of mine who has gone through miscarriage, and 7 failed rounds of IVF, recounted an occasion when a friend said this to her, the lady in question proudly cradling her own new-born at the time. Politely, my bemused friend bit her tongue, and swiftly moved the conversation along. (Such self-restraint!) Admonishing a woman quietly grieving her loss and inability to have a child, is never appropriate.

Another issue with this phrase is that it's a question of choice. Is it ever okay for a woman who has chosen to have, and subsequently been able to have, children to tell a woman who hasn't, to accept it, get over it and move on? Many would argue that unless you've been asked to impart your views or are a skilled counsellor able to handle such a conversation with expert care, it's not.

If the shoe were on the other foot even for a short while, most would struggle greatly. Again, it boils down to lack of awareness. Involuntary childlessness is a difficult grief to grasp if you've never experienced it. So it's unwise to suggest to a woman who wants, but is unable to have, children, that she should 'get over it!' Especially if she is already trying her damnedest to do just that! (Please insert your own expletives here!)

Every parent experiences supremely bad days, and is entitled to let off steam. Nevertheless, exclaiming, 'You can have one of mine!' to a woman who'd give almost anything to have children, risks being met with less than enthusiastic joviality. Some time ago, a Facebook post written by an acquaintance popped up on my feed, 'Anyone want one of my kids? Free to a good home!' Or something along those lines. In the wake of my second IVF fail, the temptation proved too much, 'Yes, I'll take one!' Naughty. I shouldn't have risen to the bait. I regret my sense of humour failure that day.

I imagine that nearly every IVF-ing woman encounters getting pregnant advice, anecdotes of miracle babies and treatment stories. I've lost count of this type of repartee: 'a friend of mine spent years trying to get pregnant, signed up for IVF, then just before they started, it happened!'. Clearly said without malice to help boost morale, but this toxic positivity is not helpful. 'Well, bully for them!' Almost teasing an emotionally fragile person into false hope days before the whole shebang is about to kick off is counterproductive, especially from a mental health perspective! Despite my better judgment, I clung to those stories every flipping time just before embarking on treatment! Only to have my tenuous hopes dashed. If there were so many bloody surprise last minute babies, then why wasn't such a miracle happening for us?

'It'll happen!' 'Try not to think about it so much.' 'Have you tried...?' 'Be grateful for what you've got!' are all in my room 101 of hapless phrases. My personal bête noire was, 'At least you've got your stepdaughter!' When uttered, I always associated this with a big pair of muddy wellies stomping all over my wish to have a child.

The implication that being a stepmother should be enough for me, perhaps I should just be grateful for that, was crass and misguided. Aren't I allowed to want my own children? My stepdaughter is one of the most important and cherished people in my life. But the desire to have my own son or daughter as well, is more than perfectly reasonable.

This does not make me greedy, nor ungrateful for what I already have. Any suggestion to the contrary is plain callous.

I've saved the best, or in this case, worst, for last. The biggest boo-boo was adoption. After our IVF fails, there were few conversations worse than those starting with, 'You can always adopt.' This phrase trips easily off the tongue. Whilst the intention must be to offer hope, I can't think of a single time that it did. I've never met a woman or man who, after experiencing fertility related loss, has been made to feel good by this remark.

Personally, I think it's akin to saying, 'What's your problem? Chin up! You'll get over it. You've still got options! Adopt a child instead.' I lost count of the times this was flippantly said as if it were a fantastically simple solution. (Just pop to the adoption shop, and select one off the shelf!) I felt like saying, 'Gosh! Why didn't I think of this before? And here I am still plugging away at my silly fertility treatments! Doh! I'll just adopt. Easy peasy. Problem solved.' (And then applying some clear gesticulations to further enhance my point!)

Whilst adoption is a wonderful way to have a family, it doesn't automatically erase the painful sadness of being unable to have your own child. Adoption isn't a one-stop-shop remedy. It's not an easy, magical fairy-tale ending. In reality, it's a huge decision, and a challenging mental, emotional, practical and financial (especially if adopting from abroad) journey in itself.

The application and adoption process is lengthy, complicated, personally intrusive, and doesn't guarantee a child, or happy family at the end of it. Suggesting adoption to couples who are likely already overwhelmed and bereaved isn't appropriate as an off-the-cuff comment or in-depth conversation unless they've brought it up themselves, or you know they feel comfortable discussing it.

So, if some people give you that crunch feeling or set alarm bells ringing when they open their mouths, I recommend you extract yourself from conversation or unnecessary interaction with them as quickly as possible. You aren't being unkind. It's simply a matter of self-preservation, establishing safer personal boundaries and practicing self-compassion. The Side-Step Strategy as I call it, comes in very handy when dodging potentially harmful conversations. I was terrible at this at first, but over time I've learnt to trust my intuition better.

How can others feel sure of what can be safely said? Well, be aware, gentle, patient, empathic and kind. Kind words can have a magical immediate impact on a person's whole day or even week. Whereas, an ill-thought out quip or dismissive gesture can send an already fragile mind into a spiral of self-doubt and anxiety.

How we speak and communicate with others really is a reflection of the people we are. I was listening to a podcast the other day, about this very topic. In it, Deepak Chopra was discussing the impact and power of our words, *'Language creates reality. Words have power. Speak always to create joy'*. Let's always try to use our words to bring joy, or at least be an alleviating salve to the hearts and minds of others. It takes practice and self-awareness, but it's possible.

I'm still learning how to think before I speak and the impact my words (and actions) might have. Sometimes, it's best to listen and offer friendship rather than lecture a person, imparting our own opinions on their precarious situation. Knowing that a person doesn't judge us, but is walking quietly alongside us, ready to catch us when we stumble, is all the encouragement, reassurance and support one might need.

Dead daft comments

PPKx-19Hzd

'You what?' I'd said,
before I punched her in the head,
whereupon she fell down
and rolled over. Dead.

Now you might think I'm crazy
or perhaps an assassin,
but there is a good reason
why I did this poor lass in!

She made a daft comment,
in fact two or three.
So I figured why not,
she's far meaner than me!

She said, 'Take it easy.
Don't think about it!'
She said, 'Put your feet up,
buy a fertility kit!'

She continued to talk.
She just waffled on.
As if the solution was simple
and I'd been getting it wrong.

'It'll happen when you least
expect it, just wait and see.
Be grateful for what
you do have and enjoy being free!'

She made me feel ungrateful.
Ashamed for feeling sad.
Like I should jolly well pull my socks up.
I felt stupid, upset and mad.

Another helpful catchphrase,
'It will happen to you one day.'
But how the heck does she know
if the 'will' will find a 'way'?

'You know my cousin Lisa?'
She went on to say.
'Well, she's got seven children now
after her initial 'delay.'

'Early nights and bedroom gymnastics.
She used to stand upon her head!'
(I know she thought she was helping,
but I'm not surprised that now she's dead!)

She offered me some special teas
and other apparent cures.
She made it sound so easy,
but I've heard it all before.

Still blabbing on about reiki, yoga,
acupuncture, and a bunch of other stuff!
I've tried them all. They didn't work.
I've really had enough!

She kept on merrily chit chatting
as if her remedies were the best.
I simply wanted her to hug me
and acknowledge the unfairness of my test.

I really needed kindness,
a little empathy,
not a know it all's approach to life,
I needed understanding and TLC.

I've had enough of being given advice
from folk who've no idea
how difficult this predicament is.
How it triggers confusion, shame and fear.

So, just be aware, dear friends (and foe)
when you utter a flippant comment,
the reality of this issue means
you're just adding to our torment.

This lass has learnt an important lesson
unfortunately, she's now splat upon the floor.
I'll prop her up in just a minute
behind the staffroom door.

If only she'd given a bit more thought
to the 'advice' she had to offer.
Do I feel guilty? Well, a teeny bit,
but at least she didn't suffer!

CHAPTER 11
Unexpected failure

'All it takes is a beautiful fake smile to hide an injured soul and they will never notice how broken you really are.'

~

Robin Williams

Not everyone can or does take time off work for the Two Week Wait. My consultant recommended that I did. This will be the recommendation for those with physical or stressful jobs. My work was both. Still commuting daily between the two sites of my split site school, two and a half miles apart, was draining. Lugging books, resources and a laptop up and down stairs to multiple rooms, weaving my way through hordes of boisterous teenagers, was physically demanding. As advised, I took a week off, combining it with a half term holiday to rest, avoiding anything that might jeopardise a successful result. My ultimate goal? Keep the embryos alive! If it didn't work, I wanted to look back without regret knowing I'd done everything I could.

Whilst waiting, I took care of my body and mind; going for walks, eating healthily, trying to have lots of sleep, staying hydrated and avoiding stressful environments. The Two Week Wait is mentally tough. Staying busy, but having a healthy balance is key. I didn't want to be twiddling my thumbs slowly going round the bend, so I wrote a journal, cooked, read, spent time with family, listened to music, and tried not to worry.

What I didn't do was spend time with friends. As the treatment had approached, and during the TWW, I withdrew significantly from my peers. I still don't fully understand the psychology behind that. I would do things rather differently now. But I battened down the hatches and propelled myself forward mainly with the help of my husband and mum. Besides, many friends were busy with new babies and toddlers. Not something I could manage to be part of during that phase.

Our consultant recommended a fertility hypnosis CD which a few times, we listened to at night to visualise the embryos growing inside me. We'd read about the power of the mind, and visualisation techniques. A couple of books described how visualisation triggers positive hormones and synapses which reduces stress helping to instil a sense of calm and empowerment.

Calm and empowerment? Yes, please! Reports by prominent psychologists outline how visualisation can improve physical and mental health. Zita West, the renowned fertility expert, recommends using such techniques to support the IVF process. It can be a powerful tool. Perhaps we'd be able to influence a positive outcome ourselves.

If you're interested in learning more about 'How The Mind Can Heal Your Body' then I recommend David R Hamilton's book of this title. What and how we think influences our bodies. It's scientifically proven that our thoughts and mind can help to heal and nurture our bodies to a certain extent. He says, '... *our thoughts even change the structure of our brains and that they send chemicals from the brain throughout the body, where they interface with cells and even DNA. We also now know that when we focus on a part of our body, the area of the brain that governs that part gets activated and the body part is activated too. And through this connection, when we visualise healing, healing occurs'.*[11]

Harnessing the power of the mind to help create a baby? Sceptical, we gave it a go, reasoning that if this type of psychological coaching was good enough for top athletes and mental strategists such as Serena Williams and Muhammad Ali, then we should at least try it. Except instead of aiming for a major tennis victory or boxing triumph, we would coach ourselves to an IVF grand slam. I made myself believe it could happen! Not every night or all the time, but I did picture them in my womb, alive. Then born and in our arms, our longed-for babies.

It may sound daft but, much like a coach spurring on the team from the side-lines, like a teacher gently urging on their weary students, like a gardener whispering to tiny shoots in the greenhouse, we often spoke to our embryos before we went to sleep, willing them to implant, put down sturdy, strong roots and grow. We were hardly maniacal about it, but if anyone had heard me wittering away to my swollen stomach in the dead of night, perhaps it would've seemed absurd and a step too far. Not to us though.

A quick word of warning before continuing. If you're tucking into a lovely meal, particularly something in a thick, rich tomato sauce, it might be prudent to put this book to one side until you've finished! An account of IVF failure wouldn't be accurate if it didn't mention the shocking amounts of blood that suddenly, like a river bursting its banks, gushes from one's body. Periods aren't great at the best of times. When it comes to IVF they're worse.

Being a woman is tremendously cruel in this regard. Reeling from shock, then coming to terms with heart-breaking disappointment is hard enough without a body that insists on brutally emphasising the point. The pregnancy test the clinic had provided was totally redundant. There was no doubt. For days, thick, dark, clotted blood flowed. My uterus was a volcanic, pulsing orb expanding and contracting like angry, clashing tectonic plates, shedding the layers of viscous tissue that the progesterone pessaries had built up for the embryos. The non-existent embryos.

My sore ovaries, the size of tennis balls, jangled when I walked. My swollen and distended abdomen throbbed and spasmed. My eyes and head ached from uncontrollable crying that came and went in waves without warning. My chest ached. I was so sad that it caused physical pain. I'd never felt so awful. Even months (in all honesty even years) later, I could still spontaneously erupt into tears despite all the effort I subsequently made to 'get over it'. I carried around a dull weight in my solar plexus that I got used to, but wouldn't completely go away.

Most fertility experts agree that the emotional and physical aspects of IVF failure are similar to miscarriage. Whilst the prospective mother has never been pregnant per-se or heard their child's heartbeat, the grief one feels is intense, raw and surprisingly traumatic. It's the loss of a longed-for child. When speaking of the psychological impact of failed treatment, particularly an unexpected failure, many couples describe feeling completely unprepared emotionally for dealing with a negative outcome alone.

Despite losing our embryos, we weren't given phone numbers for counsellors, useful support contacts, help groups, nor advice. Oddly, there was zero referral. We'd paid our money. It hadn't worked. That was that. We just kind of staggered off into the distance to deal with the emotional fallout ourselves. Without the support of the clinic. Without the support of any healthcare professionals.

If we'd known then what we know now, we would've been more assertive in seeking support. We wouldn't have flailed around in that stodgy quagmire of confused sadness. Had we had the support that we'd needed, I'd have been able to establish a proper self-care routine for us both, been more self-compassionate, and less self-critical of the fact that we were finding our life together difficult. And I'd have set more boundaries within certain areas of our lives. If we'd found help sooner, it would've made a big difference.

I've briefly mentioned the importance of preparatory care, and lack thereof. Proper aftercare in the event of treatment failure is just as essential. Whilst there are usually a couple of counselling sessions thrown in with the treatment package, it's doubtful that so few would be able to fit the brief. One or two 50-minute 'chats' is unlikely to be enduringly effective for traumatised patients.

Given the sums of money that couples spend in clinics, and considering the psychological impact that repeatedly losing embryos has, it's a meagre gesture. None of our post-IVF counselling sessions were helpful. If anything they were rather awkward, strained encounters that made us feel worse. The first, particularly so. Again, more on this shortly.

Still full of hormones after the drawn-out stress of waiting, the avalanche of feelings, shock, confusion, self-blame, loss, and anger can be overwhelming. It's an aftermath that tests the most robust of constitutions and relationships. Studies show that in the months after failed treatment, many couples experience related mental health issues. Women especially are at an increased risk of developing anxiety and depressive disorders. It's not just women of course, but we are the most vulnerable group, especially without immediate support or counselling.[12]

Men and women often have different approaches when managing tricky emotional situations. Women can be more expressive, preferring to talk and release emotions. Whilst men have more difficulties sharing their feelings. My husband falls into this category. It took him years to acknowledge how our infertility and repeated IVF failures had affected him. The cumulative effect of unresolved, undiscussed, demanding and emotionally impactful challenges had a dramatic and damaging effect on him down the line. Almost destroying our marriage.

Coaxing someone, like my husband, into talking about how they truthfully feel requires expert skill. After each failed treatment, my husband grew less emotionally communicative than usual. After the first, as I was so preoccupied myself, I didn't realise until years later how deeply he'd been affected too. Just because someone isn't crying or doesn't say they're sad, doesn't mean they aren't.

Watching me struggle to return to normal life, not being able to fix our problem, he since said, made him feel terribly guilty and powerless. He felt misled by the clinic who he too thought had done little to prepare us for our negative result. Throughout the whole process everyone had been so positive. Amazing quality eggs, great embryos, etc. He was as shocked as I was.

Yet, the only time I saw him cry was when we realised it hadn't worked, sobbing in each other's arms in our kitchen. After that, he felt obliged to be 'the strong one'. He rarely talked about the IVF. However, repressing one's feelings long term is hardly ever helpful. Bottling it up won't solve anything. Feelings find a way to surface sooner or later. In different ways, both my husband's and my own eventually did.

There's nothing in there

Numb. Undone. Disbelief.
Paralysis of stunned, raw grief.
Pounding chest. This can't be real.
The ultimate test. This wasn't the deal.

Trembling devastation.
Disorientating realisation.
'Stay strong. Hide how you feel.'
Urging myself to push through the ordeal.

Disillusion. Feeling cheated.
Confusion. Emotionally depleted.
Burning despair thinly concealed.
Unjust! Unfair! Anger revealed.

Despondency. Physical tension.
Virtual insanity. Brittle apprehension.
Blotting out pain with nerves of steel,
full of self-blame. My fate's now sealed.

Hopelessness of nowhere to hide
causes joylessness, like being dead inside.
Withered dreams flex and reel,
extinguished by the grotesquely surreal.

Lonely isolation stifles stillness.
Only desolation fills this emptiness.
Battling nausea of life without appeal,
nights of insomnia wrestling the unreal.

Oppression. Suicidal darkness.
Depression. My body a rotten carcass.
Soul stripped bare. How will I heal?
Gasping for air. Still shoulder to the wheel.

CHAPTER 12
Balancing both scenarios

'It is very hard to put into words the complexity of emotions that infertility and being a stepparent evoke in you. I would say it's constant waves of extreme ups and downs.'

~

Sarah Ironside

Have you ever been tempted to shove your head under a pillow in a darkened room, hiding until everything horrible evaporates? I was. Another regular fantasy was to take my passport from the drawer, turn up at the nearest airport, choose a random destination and buy a last-minute ticket to a far, flung land. Preferably, somewhere warm and idyllic with beautiful sandy beaches and crystal clear waters. I'd then set myself up as a barmaid living out the rest of my days in this carefree paradise. (I watched the film 'Shirley Valentine' in my youth many times. Pauline Collins is great as the downtrodden, unappreciated housewife escapee. It's still one of my favourite bittersweet comedies. If you haven't seen it, do!)

But hiding or running away is not the answer. We've got to keep going on our own paths. We've got to find a way to join in again. After each IVF failure, I resumed as near to normal life-functionality as I could. In public, I usually managed to hold things together. Sometimes though, it was pretty obvious that something was amiss. For instance, when a small baby was unexpectedly produced for show and tell, I'd perform my mute, reactionless zombie routine, followed by tears at home, comforted by my worried husband. Urgh! It was exhausting for both of us.

The trigger wasn't self-pity or jealousy. It was disorientating sadness that bubbled up from my little trauma trove. That tight ball residing in my chest. For the first few months after our first and second IVF fails, and after that on occasions when we'd just returned my stepdaughter, going to events where I'd be in close proximity to small children was excruciating. I'd get so wound up beforehand, worrying about making a spectacle of myself and how I'd feel afterwards, that sometimes I wouldn't be able to go at all.

Once again, the wisdom of hindsight and experience teaches us a powerful lesson. Had I been kinder to myself, accepted my limitations, and altered my approach, a lot of heartache, stress and mental self-flagellation could've been avoided! Explaining gently and carefully to a host that though I'd love to, I wasn't able to go, would've been a more honest and helpful strategy.

Perhaps by being more truthful, those around me would've had more insight into what was going on and how I was coping, or not, and therefore would've been able to offer a greater level of support. Covering up how we really feel makes it decidedly tricky for our friends, families and support networks to understand that a) we need their help, and b) how to help. In answer to those who cared about me who asked, 'How are you?' Instead of replying with the standard, 'I'm fine,' it would have been more helpful to have said, 'You know what, I really need a hug today'.

Establishing boundaries and having realistic expectations of myself would've been less draining. It would've also saved sufficient energy for our precious family time with my stepdaughter. Neither she, nor time with her, was stressful. Far from it. I loved it. But at weekends and school holidays, when I needed to regroup, rest and recover physically and mentally, I couldn't. Each time straight from IVF fail to busy stepmother of an energetic, bubbly little girl. From one to the other in matter of days. Adding to the steadily building pressure on our relationship.

After our first two IVFs, my husband and I no longer prioritised quality time together to properly process our trauma and loss. Life was constant 'energy out', and not much 'energy in' to refuel our depleted tanks. We both ran on empty for a long time. It's quite remarkable how so many of us manage to live like this for so long without going completely bonkers, becoming ill or having relationship breakdowns.

Whilst I'm on the subject, I must whole-heartedly make the following recommendation. If, after the whole IVF palaver, you're still in the black bank balance wise, or even if you're not and have to borrow in the short term, in my experience and that of many others, and at the advice of relationship experts, it's wise to carry out a relationship health check.

I advise a long, uninterrupted weekend away together, especially partners who've both worked throughout the Two Week Wait. Not only does this give our bodies a chance to heal and recalibrate, and our minds an opportunity to rest and disconnect, very importantly it gives our relationships much needed time, attention and space. Space to have a breather and 'just be' without IVF, trying to conceive, and external pressures. Without everything else that life throws at us.

I'm an advocate of protected 'me' and 'us' time. Relationships need space, effort and nurturing to stay on an even keel at the best of times, during the worst it's even more critical to prioritise this. No matter how caring, strong, and communicative the partnership, everyone would undoubtedly benefit from quality uncompromised time to rest, talk, and just 'be' together.

After each of our treatments, it took months for me to fully recover physically, especially after the Ovarian Hyperstimulation Syndrome. For weeks afterward, I was uncomfortable. My distended sore abdomen was awkwardly mistaken for a pregnant belly by a smiling, congratulating lady as I shuffled around our local garden centre days after our treatment fail. (That one measured highly on the Richter scale of stomach lurches for both of us, I can tell you.) Gradually, my abdomen deflated. Gradually, the hormones left my system.

Meanwhile, I focused on other things, different projects whilst we mulled over a second round of treatment. My wonderful in-laws had generously offered us the funding, but in the immediate aftermath of the first, I couldn't bring myself to think about it, let alone do it. It'd been so exhausting that I needed a break from trying to conceive, IVF, babies, or any child related subject. But when you teach small children, have many friends and family with small children and are a stepmum to a small child, you can't just bow out of the arena until you're 'ready'. Though tempting, I couldn't just 'Shirley Valentine' it off into the sunset.

The non-negotiable, transient nature of my stepdaughter's presence in our life; intense time with her, saying goodbye, having to ingloriously wait outside in the car whilst my husband took her inside, not seeing her, having no contact in between visits, then repeating the cycle, had side effects.

Each time, the suppressed child related emotions rose to the surface. It was like picking at a sore. A wound that couldn't fully heal, and a clash of feelings. The joy of stepmotherhood. Deep loss. Persistent longing for my own child. Repeat. I tried to keep a lid on it. When we were together, the three of us were a family, a unit. Our home, her second home. Our primary objective was for her to feel loved and happy.

Seeing my husband with his daughter was bittersweet. Watching their relationship grow from strength to strength, I was proud and in admiration of their beautiful father-daughter bond. Yet simultaneously, it caused sorrow. I wasn't like them. No matter how amazing I was as her stepmum, she was not my daughter in the same way that he was her dad. At times, I found this very hard. I wanted what they had. I longed for what was being tantalisingly dangled just out of reach. I wanted what I'd been told would be difficult for me to achieve. Seeing them together could cause physical pain.

An example of this paradox springs to mind. One warm summer's day, when my stepdaughter was five years old, as she was playing in our local outdoor children's splash park, she slipped and fell. Ricocheting through the air, her blood-curdling shriek caught the attention of everyone in the busy pool. All the mums and dads looked on in concern. My natural visceral response was to rush over, scoop her up and comfort her, but my husband was already on the scene.

Firstly, why did I experience such a pull to comfort her even though my husband was doing a fantastic job, especially when ordinarily the sound of a wailing child is akin to nails down a chalkboard? Secondly, why before my husband arrived on the scene, had her sobs for 'Mummy' which only lasted a few seconds, but felt like a lifetime, caused such a stomach crunch? Why did it hurt not to be the one she instinctively called for?

My friend, Sarah, recounts a strikingly similar scenario with her stepson, *'I can remember my stepson falling over and rushing to him, but him not wanting me and how that cut me to the core as I realised that I might never be anyone's fixer or first choice of comfort'*. For us both, these scenarios had a lasting impact. Our experiences as stepmothers trying to conceive our own children have certainly mirrored each other's. When feeling less than confident in my abilities and in myself, this has given me comfort and reassurance. Even now, what seems a whole lifetime later, reading her account, reminds me that I'm normal!

I do understand why some stepmothers feel threatened by their partners' existing children. When there's a strong bond, the love between a biological parent and child is unique, a third party can feel excluded. But have I ever been resentful? Never. Did I ever feel insecure? Sometimes. Was I ever overwhelmed by a surge of conflicting, confusing feelings? Regularly. The intensity often consumed me.

If this resonates with you, get yourself to a good counsellor. Don't wait like I did until you're driven half loopy. It's perfectly natural to find balancing both scenarios difficult, and normal to need support. I was out of my depth trying to reconcile grief, anxiety and anger of infertility with stepmotherhood responsibilities and feelings, while alluringly observing what I longed for between my husband and his child.

Yo-yo other mother

This daughter is a blessing,
a precious gift of life.
Chubby faced babe
to giggling girl.
One day a strong woman,
leader, mother, perhaps a wife.

Full of such potential,
exciting possibility.
As she passes through
each stage of youth,
I glimpse the woman
she may one day be.

Her natural gifts are blossoming
with encouragement and praise.
I guide her through
the toughest times,
tears and tantrums.
Still she shines light into my days.

This baby girl really loves
cuddles and bedtime stories.
And despite an independent,
stubborn streak,
needs tender
reassurance when she worries.

I pick her up, we count to ten
when she's grazed
an elbow or a knee.
I sing to her,
ride bikes, climb trees,
put on fashion shows and funny plays.

Her energy is boundless,
such a complex, clever girl.
She's quick to learn,
compassionate.
Her true character
has started to unfurl.

This child doesn't
share my DNA.
She was not created in my womb.
I did not give birth,
nor give her life.
But I'm a mother in a different way.

Yes. I am mother
of the school holiday.
Parent at weekends.
I organise her
summer trips
and Easter stays away.

At parent's evening, I'm not there,
nor Mother's day, nor nativity.
I exist behind
the scenes
in perpetual
invisibility.

For some, this routine
isn't an easy way to function.
Yet we adapt,
get on with it,
as if they were
our 'real' children.

Some long for daughters of our own,
a child we get to keep.
One that doesn't
come and go
causing sadness
even when we sleep.

Come what may we give a lot
to raise these children as our own,
often without
acknowledgement
of the care given
in the hidden second home.

Undeterred, we're fiercely proud
of all we quietly achieve.
Us, yo-yo, 'part-time,'
other mothers,
loving children
we did not conceive.

CHAPTER 13
Grandma

'I learnt a lot about my daughter, her courage, her resilience and her determination. I also learnt that the pain you feel for yourself is magnified when the pain you feel is your child's.'

~

Sally Williams

Dearest Lorna,

I'm writing to tell you how proud you make your father and I, and how sorry we are for the heartache you've endured. We've often wondered why you've had to go through this. As a parent, as a mother, it's hard to watch your child struggle, unable to take away her burdens. I've wished countless times to be able to make it happen. I've felt so powerless to change your situation.

You stay so strong and determined, so compassionate and positive, even though married life hasn't been straight forward for either of you. I'm proud too of how you've supported each other. When you were small, we knew you'd grow into a strong woman. We look at you now, and still see that same remarkable spirit, a beautiful person inside and out. Please, don't doubt that.

Every month for years, my own hope and disappointment for you alternated. A spike of optimism. Then that sinking feeling. But I told myself, 'No, that's no help. Think positive! Stay strong, and keep encouraging them.' I've always tried to be by your side whenever you need me. I trust that this is still the case. And Jon, he hides it well, but we see how much he worries about you. He looks so tired. As a mother-in-law, you don't want to intrude where it may not be wanted, but I sense he has appreciated my involvement. He has expressed that he's been encouraged by our regular small chats. It's not much, but I'm always here for him too as a listening ear, to advise, or just give a hug.

When you decided on IVF, my hope was renewed. I was glad to accompany you to appointments when Jon couldn't. Listening to the information together, it was a good option as it works for so many. I wondered how best I could support you during this stressful time. Whether you needed to call in the middle of the night or come round in person, I resolved to be available 24/7.

I was cautious when I asked how you were feeling. It's difficult isn't it? You don't want to suddenly bring up THE subject out of the blue, but then again, you don't want not to ask. Often, I waited until it felt right as you needed time and space to switch off from it all. Oh, my dear child, I've observed how all-consuming IVF is, and the toll each round has taken on you both.

Finding out your first treatment hadn't worked came as a huge shock. With every negative, waves of disappointment and sadness rolled over me, especially the first, when everything had seemed so positive. Why did it fail? My worries, frustrations and anxieties for you increased.

I was in awe of how you hid it behind a bright smile and contented demeanour telling the world you were fine, but I know you well and knew the truth. You are an accomplished actress at gatherings where babies abound. To this day, I watch you circulate at these events laughing and chatting, but I know it can still cause you pain. After each IVF, I knew that later in private there'd be emotional repercussions from putting on a brave face. I felt an ache for you.

I still feel it. Even now, it surprises me how quickly pangs of sorrow can leap up when faced unexpectedly with a new-born. As you know, I'm told that I'm a level-headed, sensible, calm person. You tell me so yourself. I hadn't expected these emotions. It's only a fraction of what you've been feeling on almost a daily basis for years, but I see just how difficult and inescapable the whole thing is. I wish I could do more to shield you from this hurt.

When anxiety began to affect your sleep, I encouraged you to keep talking. Not bottle it up. I sensed you were able to relax more after our late evening conversations. Those chats seemed to dilute your fears leading to a more restful night. You have many friends, but I understood your hesitancy to share the real extent of your struggles. I knew you feared spoiling what was a happy time for many of them, having new babies of their own. Sweetheart, even close friends find it so difficult to understand the depth of this ache. I'm glad to see that your closest friendships have withstood this toll. And that now you have such a wonderful network of supportive friendships that, if anything, have strengthened over the subsequent years.

Then there's your instinctive and natural mothering of your stepdaughter. I really don't know how you do it on top of everything else. Your strength of character is quite incredible. Your ability to stepmother, putting aside your own troubles, never letting it get in the way, is selfless and amazing. Your relationship with her is very special, so close. But I know that this came at a cost. Your parting was so very hard for you to bear. Again, I felt your sadness, adding yet another agonising layer to the loss you already carried.

I feel privileged to be involved in her life. I've never felt any resentment from her biological grandparents, but I've tended to feel that as 'just' a stepgrandmother, I shouldn't tread on her 'real' grandma's toes or overstep an unspoken, invisible line. Is this oversensitive, or tactful and cautious? I'm not sure. Not being involved in her upbringing, however, would be impossible. Though she's not your biological child, she is our family. She is loved. The gaping hole she leaves when absent is felt by me too. We all readjust until the next visit. What a complex, unexpected situation. A rollercoaster of emotions to settle back down each time. Especially for you.

As the years passed, despite your resilience, I saw the toll it was all taking on your mental health. I worried. Should we pay for regular counselling? Would this strengthen you to cope in our child centred extended family and society? Sweetheart, there's no shame in seeking expert help in these matters. It was a wise and timely decision to get help. When you started your sessions with the psychotherapist, your Dad and I quickly started to see the benefits. We were relieved.

Recently, when your Nanna rang to tell us that her 13th great grandchild had arrived safely, I felt a mixture of emotions. Great, good news! Healthy baby. Then, a lurch of pain. I can't avoid that pang, 'Ok. Let's not dwell on it, let's move on!' I told myself. I can't let myself dwell on what might, and what should've been for you too. It doesn't get us anywhere. My dear sister-in-law, grandma for the 5ᵗʰ time, wouldn't text or call me herself because perhaps she feels uncomfortable, or awkward telling me directly. Maybe she's also trying to spare our family from yet more baby announcements.

You know I don't do Facebook. Sheer self-preservation! I'm aware that there'll be a multitude of new baby pics shortly on display. Par for the course these days. Sharing photos can be good. But not appropriate for me to have regular reminders of our own contrasting family situation. I don't know how you manage it with all those baby photos popping up! Perhaps an added unforeseen bonus of moving to foreign shores is that now we're spared christening, baby shower and toddler birthday events.

Although on many levels I'd love to attend, emotionally speaking we're off the hook in that regard. I feel guilty writing this. So shortly, I'll paint a beautiful, watercolour card, congratulating your cousins, 3rd time parents, thus proving I'm not a grumpy, old sod which I fear they may think I am. I know in reality that's not their opinion, but sometimes I do wonder.

When I return to the UK next week, I'll almost have to give your aunty the go-ahead, to talk about her new grandson. I don't begrudge her. I empathise completely with how you've often described feeling, happy for a friend, but an outsider. Unavoidable. Like you, I've often felt guilty at almost having to manufacture my pleasure when the room is full of babies and toddlers and their happy parents. Your father finds it difficult too. He distances himself from it all - his coping mechanism. He grows even quieter and more distracted than usual!

When you used to come around in tears, he emotionally shut down. He couldn't bear to see your distress. He has experienced that pinch of anguish, sometimes caused too by the words of others. He remembers an unguarded comment from his aunt and godmother that should no male grandchildren be born to his children, the family line will be 'wiped out'. I know she didn't mean anything hurtful by it, but how cheery is that! As we often say when we talk, people say the strangest things.

For many in our generation, the Christmas tradition of letters from friends is an important means of keeping in touch. But as I collect each one from the doormat, I can predict the contents of most; the latest grandchild count, lovely family snapshots, babysitting to be done, another pregnancy announcement. Hey ho! I can't really be honest about our family's struggles. No one wants to know. No one knows what to say. So obviously, I've never included our delicate, and difficult family challenges in our newsletters. I don't want to be all doom and gloom. I've always skirted around the issue to avoid friends' embarrassment or discomfort. Besides, it's private. I know you've mixed feelings about who we tell. So, even face to face, I still keep many of our family updates largely to myself.

I do talk to my closest friends though. I need to talk to someone other than just your Dad to release pent up frustration and sadness. My dear friend, who herself as you know, has experienced personal loss, doesn't mention her four grandchildren until I ask and request to see photos. With her, it's never awkward nor upsetting. For some reason, I cope well with their news now they're post pre-school age. Interestingly, once children are that little bit older, it's less painful to have in-depth discussions about their progress. Why is this?

As my best friend isn't a grandmother, she's a safe haven. Our conversations are of an entirely different nature. We relax together in the knowledge that our emotions won't be suddenly challenged by a grandchild anecdote. She always asks after you, sincerely wanting to know how you and your brother are. She always asks how I am, understanding how your struggles affect me. It's a relief to keep her fully in the picture without feeling that I'm being negative or self-pitying. Her friendship, interest and support is refreshing, and helpful. We all need the support of our good friends. Keep yours close, Lorna.

Generally, I feel uneasy sharing my concerns and anxieties about your troubles with others. For one, it's highly personal, and not many understand. Secondly, searching for the right phrases without sounding self-pitying is in itself an effort. I know no other women whose daughters carry this burden and thus sympathetic comments, though meant well, can be far too glib or trite. Like you, there have been occasions when I've needed to conceal emotions amongst peer group members. Energy, diplomacy, and effort are all required. This of course, adds to the sensation of being a heartless, grumpy sod, and poor friend.

Sweetheart, I want to remind you that I'll always be here for you to listen, talk, hug, and weep. To share thoughts. Also, please don't worry about money, many parents help their children, we will help with the cost of further treatment, or counselling if you need it. Please ask, and don't feel guilty.

And keep talking, even painful conversations handled gently can relieve so much tension. Remember you're not going mad. It's perfectly normal to struggle – surrounded by seemingly glowingly happy, couples is stressful for any woman in your situation. You must strive to strike a healthy balance. It's okay to decline invitations. It's okay to feel sad. This does not make you a bad person. Never forget how special, remarkable and courageous you are.

We're so proud of you.
With love,

Mum (and Dad)
xxx

Not a grumpy old sod

QmiEimKblf

3am lying awake,
worrying about my child,
She came round again this evening,
fell into my arms and cried.

I did all I could to soothe her,
stroked her hair, wiped away her tears.
Her pain doesn't seem to lessen,
despite the passing of the years.

I'd swap places in an instant,
take her burdens as my own.
Instead all I can do is listen,
day or night, in person or on the phone

When your child is hurting,
you'd do almost anything to stop their pain,
round and round in circles,
until thinking aches your brain.

I don't know how she does it.
Few see how my daughter really feels.
Outwardly, staying positive regardless
of the heartache she conceals.

A mother knows her daughter,
a slight gesture that doesn't quite fit.
A permanent, subtle weariness
has claimed her usually lively spirit.

As a child she was adventurous,
too much independence!
I hate that this is eroding
her esteem and confidence.

This isn't what I envisaged,
but we can't guess what lies ahead.
For her, I would've chosen such a different path
from the one she has to tread.

Powerless, what more can I do
to shield her from more unhelpful knocks?
Our family needs a break
from repeated, traumatic shocks.

I've questioned myself wondering,
if it's something that I've done
that now my daughter's paying for.
A kind of cruel, twisted retribution.

Inhale. Exhale. A sigh escapes
as I consider how proud I am.
Resilience, strength, the wisdom she's shown,
coping with struggles few understand.

I fidget, moving restlessly,
too alert for sleep despite the dark.
Waiting for welcome morning light
when my anxieties won't seem as stark.

Tomorrow I'll be tired, no doubt.
Forgive me if I seem distracted.
But when my daughter suffers, I do too
through this anguish we're connected.

So, excuse me when I'm slow to smile,
less exuberant, or hesitant in my replies.
I won't have my usual energy
to keep it compartmentalised.

Our contrasting familial concerns
are at opposite ends of the scales.
I'm like a disorientated stranger in
a land of baby laden females.

If I do come across as distant, aloof,
indifferent, or vaguely odd,
please understand that it's just so tough.
And I'm not really a grumpy, old sod.

CHAPTER 14

Relationship strain

'A Venusian feels good about herself when she has loving friends with whom to share her feelings and problems. A Martian feels good when he can solve his problems on his own in his cave.'

~

John Gray

Infertility affects relationships, and dynamics within the immediate family. But none more so than with one's partner. Understanding better how to be kind to yourself whilst supporting each other throughout any challenging journey is essential to maintaining a healthy mind and secure relationship, not just for infertility sufferers.

For any couple experiencing any kind of ongoing difficulty or tension prioritising help and guidance from an experienced relationship counsellor or psychotherapist is a very good idea. If, for whatever reason, that's not immediately available, then reading is a good place to start. It's a kinder financial option in the first instance. In the second, reading how to keep your relationship afloat is a simple yet effective way to overcome your challenges whilst you consider professional help.

Pressing the eject button. Getting the heck away from it all does seem an attractive solution. Typical fight or flight response. (Hence my own airport fantasy!) So, I must take a moment to say this. If your relationship has managed to withstand years of struggle and loss, and you're still going strong, you have my utmost respect! You're both totally amazing!

It's an endurance test that not everyone can manage. It's sad, but true that many relationships break down for a lot less.

Fertility issues strain a relationship. It's not uncommon for fertility issues to be cited as one of the main influential factors leading to separation or divorce. A Danish study of 47,515 women in fertility treatment found that couples who experience infertility and subsequent complications of failed treatments, also miscarriages and stillbirths, are three times more likely to divorce or leave their partners. *'We can see that in the years immediately after the couple has been evaluated for infertility, they are around three times as likely to get divorced if the woman does not become pregnant and give birth.'*[13] Put bluntly, Dr. Kjaer, the lead author of this study, says *'not having a child after fertility treatment may adversely affect the duration of a relationship for couples with fertility issues.'*[14]

Well, blow me down with a feather! I wish we'd known this back then. Perhaps we would have been saved a lot of fuss and bother if we'd been more prepared. Another of my life mantras has sprung from this. Over the years, I've evolved into someone who dearly appreciates advance planning and preparation, after all, 'To be prepared is half the victory.'[15] Knowing what you're up against, what is expected of you, and then preparing thoroughly for the challenge makes a fantastically positive difference.

The older I get, the more I realise how wildly out of depth many of us are when it comes to communicating and empathising with others. I see it daily in my classroom. Our children, and adults too, are increasingly unable to resolve small disagreements amongst their peer groups on their own, or relate calmly and kindly to those with contrasting ideologies and opinions. Instead, many do the opposite, escalating minor disputes into dramatic, drawn out sagas.

An increasing amount of my time as an educator is spent stepping in to help and show young people how to listen to, respect and communicate positively with one another. Is this a phenomenon caused by our reliance on technology and social media rather than face-to-face dialogue? Or our worrying predilection for reality television, and social media influencers? Who or what is the real culprit for our diminishing respect and empathy in many communities today?

Even the most amazing, solid, 'straight out of the movies' relationships have mad moments. It's normal. We're all wonderful, incredible, unique beings, but we also have the capacity to be infuriatingly fallible, selfish, short-sighted and stubborn, especially when stressed or tired! For this reason, never mind 'Great Expectations' or 'Romeo and Juliet', I think the following publications should be on every secondary school compulsory reading list.

Containing nuggets of relatable observations and common sense advice and insights that can be applied to all kinds of relationships, not just romantic ones, John Gray's *Men are from Mars, Women are from Venus*, and Gary Chapman's *The Five Love Languages* had a big impact on me, my marriage, and indeed relationships with others. There are many recommendable publications that serve a similar purpose, but before seeking the guidance of a fantastic relationship therapist, these two were a winning formula for us.

Lecturer and relationship counsellor John Gray's famous book, *Men are from Mars, Women are from Venus*, was an international bestseller in the 90s. It explores the contrasting ways some men and women communicate, or rather miscommunicate, with each other. Whilst the psychology in the book came under significant scrutiny and criticism for its stereotypical portrayal of genders, I found it very useful, identifying with much of its content and observations. It's not for everyone, but if you've ever looked at your partner wondering if they're even from the same planet as you, then this book is more than worth a read.

Secondly, my favourite, Gary Chapman's *5 Love Languages* is said to be an equally, if not more transformative book. In it, Chapman, also a relationships counsellor and lecturer, gives guidance on how to improve our emotional connections and relationships with, and understanding of our partners and selves. Much like Gray's references to Martians and Venusians, initially Chapman's catchphrase terminology - keeping our 'love tanks full' was mildly off putting, but now I get it.

It's a great book that's been on the New York Times bestseller list for over 10 years! Apparently, through his talks and book, Chapman has transformed thousands of faltering relationships. For those who prefer easier, bite-sized reading material? *The Really, Really Busy Person's Book on Marriage* by Katharine Hill and Rob Parsons is just the ticket! A cute mini coffee table book of relationship nudges. It's a great conversation starter when guests find themselves leafing through its pages!

I've learnt so much from dipping into, I guess you'd call them, self-help, or motivational books over the years. My husband read extracts too, but more often humoured me when I read him snippets before bed. He would obligingly listen, but I'd turn to find him already unconscious. The soporific effect of my voice, and exhaustion rather than the content, I hasten to add! Just before lights out isn't the ideal time to start psychoanalysing one's relationship!

For the record, we weren't scouring these cover-to-cover in a desperate bid to salvage our marriage. The incremental impact of infertility was more subtle. We didn't realise how corrosive it was until we found ourselves in full on crisis mode, five years into our struggle to have a child. Our relationship had been under intense pressure for a long time. Like the frog in boiling water myth, when it's a creeping accumulation, we're often unaware until a critical point is reached. Slowly, pressure builds until one day you realise, 'Crikey, I've got to get out of here!' Not out of the relationship, I mean from the stresses and strains that the partnership is under.

It wasn't my fault, nor my husband's. We had different approaches to dealing with failing to conceive, the IVF losses and my stepdaughter's comings and goings. We didn't have blazing rows. Quite the opposite. We didn't talk honestly or in-depth at all about how we felt. I wanted to. I tried to. But when I did, rather than bringing us together, talking had the reverse effect. The more distant my husband became. So much so, I felt I was damaging our relationship. So, I stopped trying. I thought that like him, I should have a stiff upper lip. This led to feeling very low and alone.

Do you see the pattern? Feeling low. Needing to talk. Trying to talk. Met with apparent indifference. Feeling low. Needing to talk, etc, etc. Unhealthy. But normal. Like many couples, focusing on the practical running of our lives, rather than nurturing the emotional side of a relationship, was how we existed. (Dr Chapman would tell us to fill up our 'love tanks' immediately. We were running on empty!) To an observer though, and even to us, it was barely detectable at first. As is often the case.

Friends, families, colleagues in supportive roles need to be more aware of the strain that infertility puts on a relationship not just in the immediate aftermath, but for years afterwards. Having the right support and understanding is essential. Many couples who experience unsuccessful in vitro fertilization treatment who remain childless are still deeply affected by ongoing grief at least three years later.

The continuing impact of infertility and failed treatments is usually huge. The grieving process not only impacting a relationship in the short or medium term, but continuing for years. It's a silent grief that the marriage is constantly having to navigate and adapt to. Involuntary childlessness is an additional marital pressure. (Especially when one of the two is already a parent.)

It's hard to know when someone is grieving. We generally don't wear a t-shirt or announce it with a claxon when we enter a room. Being aware and intuitive is paramount. Take my husband, for example. Not one for displays of emotion, more the stoic type. Apart from the day we'd found out treatment had failed, he exerted extraordinary levels of self-control, never expressing his emotions openly. He has since admitted to a bout of 'letting it all out', retreating into the shed where alone, surrounded by gardening paraphernalia and bikes, he had a private weep. I had no idea.

Whilst I'm grateful for his remarkable self-restraint and strength, it would've been healthier and more helpful if he'd talked to me rather than hiding it. Talking honestly together helps a couple feel mutually supported and strengthened. Personally, it helps me to stay emotionally connected to my husband. Regularly sharing how we feel is comforting, and fundamental to the friendship side of every partnership. We need to be heard. We need to feel understood and valued by our partners. This is essential.

Male partners often feel they must be 'strong'. Yet, we know that compartmentalising and burying our worries, fears, stresses, inevitably leads to problems later. Left unaddressed, depression or grief will manifest itself, usually in harmful ways. My emphatic advice to men (and women) is not to ignore it. There's no shame in discussing feelings. Couples going through any heartache must talk. Not big whinges and moans, simple regular 'check-ins' with our partners. Asking how they're feeling. Prioritising time and space for each other, and properly listening. Responding to each other's emotional needs is vital to the survival of any relationship, and any family.

This may not come naturally. If it's not already a regular habit, it may feel odd. But if we truly love and want the best for each other, and ourselves, and want healthy, lasting relationships, effort must be made. For those who don't, sadly, leaving or blaming our partners for our stress and unhappiness often ends up being the more tempting, easier solution rather than making the effort to dig in and connect honestly with the other person. If we truly want a thriving relationship and wholesome, enjoyable family life, we must be prepared to step out of our comfort zones. As Chapman says, long-lasting, fulfilling, emotional love is a choice. We must sometimes choose to learn, choose effort, and choose love.

For my husband and I, learning to better recognise the signals and intervene when the other person was struggling was hard initially. And though he still finds it difficult to talk about emotions, particularly those related to our fertility heartaches, he tries and is far better than he was, *'At first, I struggled to understand the emotions my wife was going through. I certainly struggled with what to say. I now realise that it isn't a problem I can solve through practical solutions, I just need to understand the pain and listen. I have learnt (slowly) to express my feelings on the issue and be better at listening. In a way, it's almost like learning a new language – a language that I was far from fluent in previously'.*

We've both had to work, quite hard at times, to 'speak each other's language' in order to keep our relationship balanced and healthy. What does a healthy relationship look like? Well, I would say, one that doesn't have you in a permanent state of worry or stress. One that makes you feel good about yourself. One that brings out the best in you and your partner. And one in which you enjoy being together. One that makes you happy.

The guardian

Rb3Cq54yqd

Gazing through the window
across the damp autumn garden,
he lets out a long, deep sigh
as he stands motionless in the kitchen.

A solitary blackbird swoops in low
catching his attention
it sings out shrilly as if to him,
momentarily he forgets his apprehension.

Suddenly, the coffee splutters,
interrupting his absorbed reflection.
He switches off the machine with a frown
that betrays his lingering tension.

He adds the milk, his movements calm,
despite the knot tightening in his stomach.
He wonders how he should comfort her.
If only it were as simple as in that book.

Resolutely, he pushes back his shoulders,
picks up the mugs to take them through.
He might not be confident with soothing words,
but he resolves at least to say a few.

Seeing her changed by so much sadness,
watching her vibrancy fade away,
he hates it, she shouldn't have this burden.
He scolds himself, 'Why can't I figure out what to say?'

The lounge feels odd like it's not theirs.
A strange emptiness has sucked out all the air.
Passing her coffee, he shudders a little,
then sits softly, turning to stroke her hair.

Curled up on the sofa, she smiles at him,
it makes him want to weep.
If only he could lift her up, carry her,
but he's immobilised. He too feels so weak.

He hurries through his morning routine,
with weary, yet renewed determination.
As he cleans his teeth, he tells the mirror,
'I'll be enough for both of us'. A bit of self-motivation.

Backing out the driveway,
tyres crunch on the gravel drive,
he hesitates glancing at the house
backlit by a dreary, unpromising sky.

Despite a familiar lurch at leaving her,
he changes gear, flicks on the lights.
He runs through his list of briefing notes,
mentally composing emails he's got to write.

The chatter of the radio host accompanies
him as he continues to plan his day.
His fingers start to tap the wheel
as his favourite song begins to play.

An idea takes shape in his already full mind.
Emotional stuff may not be his thing,
but he'll book them a surprise hotel treat.
He'll find a good deal this evening.

The traffic has eased. He's almost there.
Relieved, he no longer feels so conflicted.
A break together that will help.
He feels better. His morning gloom has lifted.

CHAPTER 15
Multi-layered loss: feckless father

'I'm still practising, I'm still learning, still getting corrected in terms of how to be a fine husband and a good father. But I will tell you this: everything else is unfulfilled if we fail at family, if we fail at that responsibility.'

~

Barack Obama

Before I came on the scene, my husband was an expert in repressing and compartmentalising feelings. He had quite a few locked away. His routine and emotional life after the birth of his daughter continued to have an impact on our relationship years later. To manage his lifestyle effectively back then, his emotions were locked down, subsequently becoming such a pro that once infertility struck, he reverted to his tried-and-tested, default setting to cope without pesky emotions getting in the way! Not very helpful when you're married to someone who needs to express and talk about her feelings to feel sane!

Like rock strata, the worry, guilt and powerlessness of failing to conceive a child with me were layered atop a well-established bedrock of feelings linked to his daughter's unexpected arrival. He says that, in the short term, the ability to compartmentalise in this way was a convenient skill, *'I guess you could say that when I became a dad it helped to compartmentalise my emotions, keep the emotions tucked in. I wasn't aware I was doing that. I just did it. There were a lot of changes all at once, a demanding job, I'd just changed career. I had just bought a house, and my daughter arrived. I simply didn't have time, or mental space to think about, or over analyse emotions. I just kept calm and carried on with my responsibilities. I wasn't consciously blocking out emotions. Looking back, I had to bury certain feelings, which some can do naturally, more easily than others. It helped not to get consciously emotionally stirred up about things. I know it's not healthy long-term, but it can be a strength. I got on with my life despite the changes in lifestyle, and challenges.'*

He's quite right. After all, who has the time and energy to deal with inconvenient emotions in this busy and demanding day and age? Firstly, lifting the lid can be exhausting. Secondly, you never know quite what's going to come out when you do, or how it'll manifest itself. Thirdly, for many of us finding the 'time' to nurture our emotional selves can seem almost impossible. And finally, putting complex emotions to one side does free up mental space for other responsibilities and priorities. Keeping a lid on it can certainly appear advantageous.

However, repression does little good to either our physical or mental health in the long run. We cannot control our feelings indefinitely. Though some of us try to be, we're not machines. We are sentient creatures that must express ourselves. There's only so long we can keep it all held in. Whether we like it or not, sooner or later our emotions will demand our attention. Or our health and relationships will begin to suffer. Like water, emotions eventually find the path of least resistance to seep through. If you've seen spectacular images of cracked dam collapses, you'll be able to picture how that ends!

My husband's early experiences of fatherhood were undeniably complex and challenging. He was, by his own admission, buffeted by exhaustion, doubt and self-reproach. It's not unusual for first time fathers to experience bouts of self-doubt and lack self-esteem. Like many new parents, he questioned his efforts, hiding his worries behind a confident exterior, *'I never experienced anxiety, but I did doubt myself because I thought I wasn't doing a good enough job of everything, combining my daughter with work, and my family; trying to be good at everything at the same time, trying to multitask different roles on my own and be really good at all of them. I felt I wasn't doing well enough in any of them. I worried about my relationship with my daughter. I wanted us to be close. I wanted to see her more often, but she lived with her mum, and was just a baby.'*

Worry is normal for every parent type, but particularly so for those with more complex childcare arrangements and circumstances. The guilt and worry he felt, though understandable, was unfounded. But then, a lot of parents, it would seem, frequently berate themselves for not being a 'better' mum or dad. Many friends, over the years, have spoken of regular bouts of 'mother guilt' which seems to be endemic today in parenthood, especially motherhood, in western cultures.

Indeed, parenting can be a tough journey and learning curve regardless of the familial set up. This is exacerbated for parents who aren't with their children daily. For them there is an extra, usually unspoken or unacknowledged, element of anxiety, fear and even alienation. But there's no silver bullet for any of us when times are tough. No magic fail-safe formula for raising well-adjusted kids. We all just have to do our best, trusting that we're treading the right path with our offspring.

This is what my husband has always done. His best. The lengths and breadths to which he went, and still goes, as a father is commendable. Subsequently, he has a strong, loving and affectionate relationship with his child. Admittedly, I'm a little biased, though my observations are also based on fact and experience. I've spent a significant portion of my career dealing with the fallout of parents who do not have their child's emotional well-being as a priority.

I witness him as a consistently positive role model and balancing influence in his daughter's life, underserving of the not-so-subtle disapproval that sometimes hangs in the air between a father in his position and critics. I make this point to encourage others like him. Never having lived together full-time hasn't stopped a strong bond between them being forged.

'Thankfully, my relationship with my daughter is strong. I was, I am, immensely proud of her. The connection we had even as a baby, and still have, is one of the most important aspects, the best aspects of my life. I wanted more than anything to be a good dad, and role model. I enjoy being with my daughter, obviously, she's my child. I'm her dad. Not always living in the same household doesn't change that.' Rather than one stressful, conflict-stricken home like some of our students, his daughter has two stable, affectionate and understanding homes, which is a basic requirement for any child to develop into a well-rounded, versatile adult.

He has told me that preparing to become, then becoming a new dad was a period in his life when he felt very lonely. His own emotional needs were put to one side in order to focus on his new responsibilities, his child and helping her mum. He loved his daughter, but it was not a happy time for him. It was highly stressful and isolating.

Single dads, that is to say, dads without partners, are a statistically vulnerable group as far as mental health is concerned, *'It was hard. I missed lots of 'first' things in my daughter's life. I would've liked to have been able to experience those first-hand. I was never depressed, but worrying about her was at the back of mind, underneath things all the time, I suppose that was an extra pressure, an extra load that contributed to feeling very tired mentally. As I've said, I wasn't aware of it affecting my mental health at the time, but I now see that it did.'*

Canadian research[16] into loneliness and single fathers has found that they're much less likely to have a strong social network around them for support than single mothers. It's this absence of effective support and ensuing loneliness that, the study suggests, may be contributing factors to the increased mortality rate among single dads which is three times higher than for single mums and partnered fathers.

Three times higher! We already knew that loneliness is bad for us, but it would seem especially so if you're a single dad. As a society we're increasingly aware of (although still not as much as we should be) the challenges mums without partners often face. Dads on their own, however, are a far less understood, more overlooked and in some cases, even stigmatized group.

This loneliness study led me to wonder if post-natal depression might also be a factor for new fathers. It's not so readily associated with the male context. According to an NHS report, one new mum in ten experiences PND within the first year of giving birth. The Fatherhood Institute, the UK's leading fatherhood think tank, states that the figure is much the same for dads. Further research by the NCT in 2015 found this figure was probably much higher. One third of fathers express concerns about their mental health. Worryingly though, men who do experience mild to moderate post-natal mental health issues are far less likely than mothers to talk or receive support.

I'm not suggesting for a moment that my husband fell into this post-natal depression category. He didn't exhibit depressive symptoms. For him, it was more the corrosive impact over time of these unresolved emotions on top of which, heaped like a pile of manure, our fertility was dumped. The steaming icing on the cake!

At the time, recognising that professional help would be wise, he did have several sessions with a counsellor, but that wasn't as effective as he'd hoped, *'A good friend suggested I should see a counsellor. He saw that I was struggling with everything on my plate emotionally, and maybe from a mental health perspective. I can barely remember the counselling. I think I had so much going on, and some things were quite difficult, that I've kind of blanked it out. It's a bit hazy. I don't remember gaining anything from it, no helpful insight. It must have been quite bland not to stick in my mind. I don't think I really clicked with the counsellor either. I can't even recall what the lady looked like, if I'm honest.'*

To get the best out of talking therapy, it's essential to find a therapist who puts us at ease, and to whom we feel comfortable talking, with whom we connect, and who is helpful. Effective counselling for him didn't happen until much later.

Did you know that the whole month of November is Men's Mental Health Month in the UK? For those interested, there's a whole load of information available on the website mentalhealth.org.uk. Mental health awareness for men has vastly improved. Yet, there still seems to be a lingering stigma for men of talking to their friends and family about problems. Feeling you ought to be strong and dependable still seems imbedded in society. Judging yourself as a failure when you don't feel strong is common.

Rather than seeking help, a father with depressive symptoms is therefore more likely than not to keep up appearances for fear of being viewed as a 'bad dad' or 'weak man'. Some new fathers speak of feeling left out of the bonding process with their child, not feeling needed, having no one to talk to who understands, lacking confidence in their new role and feeling like a less important, inferior parent, and even feel insecure about their relationship with their child.

This is certainly relatable to my husband during the first couple years of his daughter's life, *'I didn't really speak about my biggest fear until my wife came along. My fear was that my daughter would be taken to Brazil, where her mum is from, and I'd have no say in that decision. Her being taken away was a thought I had a few times. I felt I didn't have control over that. Someone else could call those shots. I didn't think it would happen, but it was definitely something I thought about because you just don't know in these kinds of situations. I worried too that I'd messed up my life, my daughter's life, her mother's life. I didn't consciously worry all the time, they were thoughts that popped up every now and again. And, of course, as I've said, it all tied into the worry that I should be a better dad.'*

It didn't help that some folk, even those he knew well, made unintentionally derogatory comments. Like we've mentioned, those who temporarily forgot he was a father, 'When you have kids, you will...' The 'just a part-time' dad label didn't do much to encourage or build his self-esteem and confidence either. Anyway, if you're a good, involved and affectionate parent, I'm not sure that you can be part-time. There are certainly different types of parent, but not part-time in this context.

When 'full-time' parents are glad to see the back of their offspring for a short while, they don't stop being a parent. As a parent, you don't clock in and out of your 'shift' completely. There is usually still a heck of a lot going on emotionally speaking. For most, our minds are active, worrying or thinking about our children even when they're not physically with us. We don't stop being a family just because a child is not physically there.

'I've never regarded myself as a part-time parent. The terminology or idea of part-time isn't very helpful. There needs to be another term, another simple way of saying that you're a parent whose child doesn't live with you all the time. It's not about the amount of time you spend together. It's quality time that you spend together. If you're a good parent, you're a role-model and parent regardless, not part-time.'

'How you spend your time together is obviously important; creating lasting, positive memories, nurturing your child's interests, and helping them overcome aspects of life that they're finding difficult, being aware of how your child is feeling, and responding to that in a way that helps them. Teaching them boundaries, compassion and, (this is my wife's word) gratitude for the little things is important too. Caring and nurturing is all part of parenting, listening to them when they want to talk to you, not being too 'busy' with other things to help them. When I know my daughter feels secure, safe, and happy, I know things are ok.'

So, we shouldn't listen to those who undermine us, or put us down, those that don't include us in 'parenting' conversations, those who think they know best, because they don't necessarily. Parenting and making the right choices for our families is a learning experience for everyone. Sometimes, we totally nail it. Sometimes, we fall flat on our faces. Sometimes, we realise how we could tweak it for next time.

If you or your partner are in a similar situation, try not to let disparaging comments about being a 'part-time' or less important parent or similar, damage your confidence or resolve. You are an intrinsic, essential part of your child's life. You are your child's family. And your contribution isn't automatically devalued just because your child doesn't live with you 7 days a week. Being a good dad or mum, or stepdad or stepmum, is not measured on whether your home is their permanent residence or not.

Empathy

'Don't judge a man until you've walked
a mile in his shoes.'
But people do they criticise,
imparting unsolicited views.

They haven't got the t-shirt,
not been through the test.
Such audacity is ballsy
to assume they know it best.

Blundering words tumble forth,
spoken out of habit.
Mean? Judging? Condescending?
They don't realise that they do it.

Or perhaps they do, to remind a man,
keep him in his place.
Strike the target where it hurts!
Devoid of empathy and grace.

Critical words have power to harm
even the strongest man!
Lacking care, kindness, self-control
it's more than some can stand!

Or just take the piss. Ha, ha. Funny.
Stick on a good-natured grin.
Is it really humour though?
The joke's wearing a little thin.

Nothing said can be just as odd.
Cool as ice indifference.
No words of comfort, no acknowledgement.
A wall of remote silence.

Skirting round the elephant
wedged enormously in the room.
When no one wants to mention it,
it's kept under the carpet, schtum.

To be oblivious to the hour
of need of a fellow human being,
it can't always be so difficult
to sense how another person's feeling.

Surely empathy's not forgotten?
Not completely dead and withered?
Dig it out. Dust it off. Reach out to
those feelings that should be considered.

Let's lighten the load for those we know.
A simple, kind, well-timed gesture.
Show them that they're not alone.
Help ease the burden that they shoulder.

Let's bridge the gap. Stand together.
Make a difference in our families.
The world would be a far kinder
place with a bit more empathy.

CHAPTER 16
Multi-layered loss: mad other mother

'It's difficult for others to understand the depth of the loss we feel for the child who will never be born. Even those closest to us may wonder why we can't seem to get over it.'

~

Author unknown

Although I'm quite taken with the image of riding in as my husband's gallant rescuer, I'm not suggesting this was the case! But coming along when I did, made an immediate difference, *'Being with my wife, the three of us, was less intense, more relaxed, more fun. I had someone, to share my daughter with, rather than trudging around London on my own, feeling a bit lonely. I had friends, but I didn't really talk to them about things I was finding difficult. I found it easier to talk to Lorna. She listened, and gave me advice without being too pushy. Our relationship eased the pressure. She made me laugh more, be less serious, gave me perspective.'*

'My wife was, is, loving and caring with both of us, especially with a baby girl that wasn't biologically hers. We both felt happy when she was with us. I'd say that she helped me bring my head back above water, helped me stay afloat. I guess it felt like she buoyed me up, brought me back to feeling like me again, having been weighed down subconsciously by many different feelings. She helped me find a way to feel like me again, but also be a good dad, and partner without losing myself amongst it all. You could say, she helped me become a new, improved version of the old me.'

To this day, it feels good to have that early hard graft acknowledged and appreciated. He no longer felt so alone. The stronger our partnership became, the less anxious he felt. He had someone to talk to regularly. Mulling things over together boosted his morale. I reminded him of the ways I saw him being as fair and consistent as possible to each one of us involved in raising his daughter, and an amazing dad. Gradually, his confidence grew, and his worries though unable to disappear entirely, shrank.

It's funny how after feeling so strong, trying to help my husband, the situation soon seesawed. A role reversal. The problem was that my husband was very much out of his depth when it came to trying to help me. I think most would be when faced with your wife rolling around on the bedroom floor, sobbing, gasping for air in the middle of the night, 'You don't understand how I feel! How can you? You're already a father'. Pause. Then a bit more, 'I really fucking hate this. I feel trapped. Why can't I have my own baby? What's wrong with me? You've got a beautiful daughter. I want to be a mother. I can't keep doing this. This is cruel'. Exhausted, I would eventually cry myself to sleep

Poor, patient husband, how draining it was for him. Nights after my stepdaughter had gone were the worst. Emphasising my childlessness, it triggered grief each time. It was as if my own child had been taken away. I oscillated between sadness, rage, and acceptance.

Neither of us had ever heard anything like the animalistic noises I produced. Tremendous raging and roaring spread like wildfire. I'd writhe, wail, and swear! If I'd been holding it in for few days, like a tsunami it arrived with raw, unfettered energy from the depths of my gut. Sometimes, my sobbing kept us awake long into the night. By morning, we ached with mental and physical fatigue. The fact that were able to function at work the following day is remarkable really.

Attacks were brutal. I became another person. Jeckyll and Hyde. Calm and composed by day. A raging lunatic by night. My husband, powerless to solve the problem, didn't know how to comfort me. My outbursts semi-paralysed him. Infuriating me even more sometimes. I just needed to be held, calmed by his reassurances, and have someone close to me. I felt so alone. My own behaviour scared and confused me. After these bouts, I felt numbly empty, or was filled with shame and self-loathing. Why was I not coping better? I should be a better wife, stepmother, friend, daughter, colleague... Why wasn't I a more 'normal' human being?

It wasn't just nocturnal. Sometimes, an unfortunately timed comment or mismanaged announcement could confine me to my bed crying on and off during the day too. I cried so hard it was painful. I was barely able to function afterwards. The rest of the afternoon would be spent sleeping it off whilst my husband did his best to soothe me, brought mugs of tea, ran the house, and looked after me.

Our hybrid lifestyle kept me in a twilight zone, unable to follow suggestions 'to forget about it,' 'focus on other things,' 'have a breather just the two of you during half-term.' I didn't have that option. So much time spent in places abundant with young children every school holiday doesn't facilitate 'forgetting'! Exhaustion compounded the problem. Trapped in this cycle, increasingly dark thoughts entered my mind. I was unwell.

Suicidal thoughts aren't unusual. And sadly, infertility related suicides happen. When respondents of the 2016 *Fertility Network UK Survey on the Impact of Fertility Problems* were asked about suicidal thoughts after failed treatment, over 2 in 5 reported that they had these feelings either occasionally, sometimes, often, or all the time. I would put myself in the 'sometimes' category. Usually, when I felt utterly hopeless, I took strange, detached pleasure in contemplating different 'ways out'.

Awful. But I didn't just have these thoughts when bereft. I'd catch my mind wandering whilst watching TV, cooking dinner, driving to work, at work, after a normal conversation with a colleague... A joyless place to climb out of without psychological help. Miserable for my husband to watch his strong and rational wife deteriorate. It wasn't like this every day, but bad patches continued on and off for years.

I was genuinely pleased for other people's pregnancies, but they could debilitate me out of the blue. Conversations with strangers could trigger the knotted stomach feeling. A common culprit could be, 'And do you have children?' Lurch, hot flush, panic. Was it shame? Awkwardness, in case there was a tricky follow up question? Or fear of more tears later? This question is merely asked to get conversation going, find common ground, or be polite. When you're married, of childbearing age, and because child chit-chat is an acceptably safe topic, women tend to ask this type of thing. Men, so my husband says, not so much.

'Do you have kids?' Publicly acknowledging that I didn't, activated my solar plexus trauma trove. 'We'd like some, yes', was an option, but might lead to an unwelcome extension of the conversation. 'No, I don't,' on the other hand, wasn't truthful. Not mentioning my stepdaughter felt like betrayal. But I wasn't my stepdaughter's *real* mum. Did I count? Lacking confidence. Over analysing. Worrying. Unable to deal with what I interpreted as disapproval or judgment when they found out how young she was and jumped to their own conclusions. Often, I said nothing.

What a stew I used to get into over many things! It took years for me to talk proudly and confidently about my stepdaughter, 'Yes. I'm a stepmum!' I no longer fear those words, or the rebuff, 'Yes, but she's not *your's*,' or words to those effect which have, on more than one occasion, been said. I'm proud to tell people about her. She's a huge part of my life, and I don't care so much what is thought of me.

Anyway, I would hope that most would feel reassured and uplifted to hear a stepmother speak enthusiastically about her stepchild. To all hardworking, loving stepmothers out there, a huge shout out! Give yourself permission to be bold, proud and truthful. Don't hide what you do, or the relationship you've carefully crafted with your inherited child. When asked THE question, use it as an opportunity to enlighten others. Many of us make huge sacrifices behind the scenes, making big differences to the lives of young people. It must be acknowledged! Stepparents, let's be seen and heard!

Ok. I've climbed down from my soapbox. Back to withering self-esteem! Going out for a social event? I'd begun to dread it. Worrying how I'd cope if something 'happened'. If I had a funny turn, would I make a fool of myself? Would friends lower their voices, whisper and avert their eyes, thinking I couldn't hear their child or pregnancy conversations that I pretended not to notice? I went out less. Talked less. Isolated myself more. Although I tried to choose wisely which events would be safe and which to forgo, a handful did not end well. Slap on the smile. Wait till I got home. Collapse.

For example, one evening whilst my husband was away, exhausted and disappointed, again having built up false hope due to a late period, I needed the easy company of a good friend. I worried about going out, but it was the tonic I needed. I didn't want to be alone. Chilled out dinner and drinks with a dear childhood friend who knew my heartache. What could go wrong? When my friend came to the door to collect me, I should've said something then. Alas, I did not. I certainly didn't wish to greet her with negativity and whinges.

We didn't even make it to the restaurant before the bomb was dropped. Her words hung in the air between us as I sat frozen and mute in the passenger seat whilst she drove. My mind was screaming, 'Say congratulations, congratulate her, you half-wit!' It was so loud, I'm surprised it didn't audibly blast through my ears into the gulf between us.

Nothing happened. I said nothing. Didn't move. Just stared out of the windscreen. If I'd been a stunt woman, I would've opened the door, executed a splendid James Bond-esque kamikaze roll out of the moving vehicle, and sprinted away back up the street.

I'm not proud of my reaction. But I did the best I could at the time. In my defence, I was mentally unprepared, and just so exhausted from 'faking it' with the smile, with the 'I'm fine, thanks.' My reserves had let me down because, yes, I was 'running on empty'. No warning or gentle preamble, my guard was down. But, my friend deserved better. Pregnant with her first child, she'd wanted to share her exciting news.

Much to her relief (and mine), I finally spluttered out unconvincing best wishes, words unjumbling themselves from my 100-mile-an-hour, screaming brain, forming flat, awkward sentences. Awkwardness that followed us into the restaurant. I braced myself for an evening of keeping up appearances with a friend who knew me too well to be fooled by my stilted attempts to keep my tears at bay.

Oh my goodness, her suggestion to go back to my house for fish and chips instead was a relief! Although what I actually wanted was to put on my PJs, climb into bed, sink a bottle of vino and have a good cry. Alone! I don't know if my friend was aware how hard I found the rest of that evening. Masking and controlling my emotions not to upset her further.

What would I do differently now? Well, pretty much all of it. Our outing was doomed from the get-go. I should've been totally honest from the outset. If it had still been uncomfortable, I'd have contained the situation before it escalated and asked to postpone our evening to when I was more able to share her joy. I would've hugged her and asked to be taken home. Not in a mean-spirited way. But in an 'I know my limits' kind of way.

I've certainly learnt since then that we shouldn't keep pushing ourselves beyond our emotional limits. But as Confucius is cited to have said, '*By three methods we may learn wisdom: first by reflection which is the noblest; second by imitation which is the easiest; and third by experience which is the bitterest*'. Amen to that!

Honesty for me has always worked best. Making the effort to give a little non over-the-top, factual background with care means that it's up to others how they wish to respond. You may find that compassionate friends, able to empathise and wishing to reach out, will do all they can to support you. Popping round to check you're ok. Phoning, WhatsApping you. Bringing emergency wine when needed! Suggesting a little lunch out, or a Netflix comedy evening when they know you're feeling low.

I would advise against completely hiding ourselves away without explanation. It can drive friends away. It's confusing. Some may take it personally. Plus, self-isolation can add to the self-esteem spiral. As soon as we distance ourselves from those we love, the harder it is to combat anxieties and insecurities. We can end up more alienated from the very people we need around us.

The importance of talking is an ongoing theme throughout this book. I should've talked and asked my friends more for their help. Instead, some didn't really understand what was going on, how much I struggled and how to help. Some were confused by my detachment.

Everyone else but me

i5bCBZj2Lu

Tall ones, short ones,
waddling about.
Big bellied, rotund ones,
about to pop one out.

Ones in summer vest tops,
getting fish and chips.
Ones shuffling round Waitrose,
selecting hummus dips.

Ones who look as pleased as punch,
stroking bulging tummies.
Ones who seem not to notice
their metamorphosis into mummies.

Ones who don't seem to care,
they treat it as a joke.
Even though they're up the duff,
they still drink and swear and smoke.

Those who prattle endlessly
about their pregnancy.
Those who barely say a word,
just a comment occasionally.

Those who post it all on FaceBook,
happy selfies with their scan.
Of course, they're bloody gonna to gloat,
just because they can.

Those who are quite tactful whilst
others really aren't.
Those who bravely persevered
after being told they can't.

There's those that blossom, those that don't.
Those that vomit, ache and sweat.
Those whose skin is radiant,
they look immaculate.

Some develop OCD
tidying everything.
Others end up so chilled out,
'Who cares if nothing's clean?'

Some have names already picked out.
Others haven't got a clue.
Some are so ultra-organised
there's little left to do.

Some manoeuvre gingerly,
down the busy street.
Their ankles swell, and skins react
in the baking August heat.

Some loll around at the beach,
wearing teeny, tight bikinis.
Perfectly posed to show off
proud, protruding bellies.

Those who didn't plan their child,
didn't even try.
No need to bonk for years on end.
No little monthly cry.

Others who'd felt terribly hopeless,
they'd lost all self-belief.
They'd needed umpteen treatments
to help them to conceive.

Those whose babies started in a dish,
costing loads of smackeroonies.
Injecting drugs, and taking pills
that turned them into loonies.

Some who have a story to tell,
incredulous at their miracle.
Some still can't believe it,
they didn't think it possible.

Some whose bellies stay empty,
but who carry on regardless,
refusing to accept their bodies
will leave them completely childless.

Some who laugh, and chatter
despite an inner grief.
Infertility has robbed them.
A cruel and heartless thief.

Others see a counsellor
to talk about their pain.
It's driven them bananas.
They think they've gone insane!

Some still can't understand it.
It seems so easy for everyone else.
Others whose relationships end.
It's ruined their mental health.

Some who just get on with it,
surrounded by fertile women
whose partners clearly don't have
any issues with their semen.

Some who feel immobilised
by babies in every womb.
Others who dream of jacking it in
and moving to the moon.

CHAPTER 17
Self-esteem and depression

'Depression is the most unpleasant thing I have ever experienced... It is that absence of being able to envisage that you will ever be cheerful again. The absence of hope. That very deadened feeling, which is so very different from feeling sad. Sad hurts but it's a healthy feeling. It is a necessary thing to feel. Depression is very different.'

~

J.K. Rowling

Even in Western cultures, childlessness has a peculiar status. One can feel substandard, inferior, a spare part, an outsider. On the other hand, not having children can be liberating, rewarding; a socially and personally enriching decision. I admire those around me without children who live fulfilled, purposeful, dynamic lives, making lasting contributions to their communities. Their identity and sense of self-worth are certainly not tied up with being, or not being, a parent.

I saw this. I wanted this. I just had to flip the switch telling me I wanted motherhood. Freedom to make other life choices without being brought back to the same 'conundrum' was very appealing. I tried. But it's hard to change the wanting a child mind-set. At one stage, I contemplated hypnotherapy. Like when people want to stop smoking, I wondered if it might have a similar effect. Removing the desire for a cigarette, removing the desire for a child. Was it so different?

The social and cultural element of childlessness is interesting. Despite the progress we've made in Western cultures regarding equal rights and the role of women, there's still a long way to go, especially when it comes to motherhood. The stigma of childlessness is ingrained in the fabric of society.

The other day, I was talking to a Spanish friend whose sister had an IVF round that had failed a few years previously. The whole, large Catholic family would ask about it every time they saw the poor woman. What was happening? Any news? When was she going to have kids like her sister-in-law? What pressure! What intrusion!

Recently, her sister announced she was pregnant. The family was in a rapturous state of ecstasy! Not because it signalled an end to her sister's plight, well that too, but mainly, so my friend told me, because it was now easier for everyone. No more awkwardness. No more family shame when friends asked. Her pregnancy had bought her back into the fold, eliminating the family's social discomfort.

My friend suspects that the pregnancy was a result of more treatment, but her sister won't talk about it. Seeking Assisted Reproductive Treatment rather than conceiving naturally had caused a deep sense of shame for her the first time; a process that her family, aunts, uncles, cousins all with multiple children didn't really understand, and in some cases, fully support.

Feeling the black sheep of the family at social gatherings and events when almost every family member of your generation has a child running around or dangling from their hips, is horrible. Especially in such a family orientated Hispanic culture. Not being able to conceive naturally, should her sister have admitted to it, still would have caused an element of shame and failure. Urgh! There is so much goddamn shame associated with infertility! Until it happened to me, I had no idea how it makes you feel as a woman, how it can undermine our sense of femininity, identity and worth. Anyway, all's well that ends well for her sister!

For those of us who find ourselves on the edge of certain social parameters, let's keep a sense of perspective. It could be worse. In many developing countries, motherhood is *essential* to a woman's social position. For a childless woman, the degree of social isolation that she experiences is often life changing. Her identity, perceived usefulness, value to society is measured by whether she has children, and in some cases, how many.

Whole communities shun women unable to conceive. Women are abandoned by their husbands in favour of another wife, avoided by other women fearful that it's 'catching,' accused of witchcraft or having the 'evil eye,' prevented from attending certain social events, and even abused. Childlessness. Failure. Shame. Stigma. So toxic and destructive. Imagine being ostracised by your entire community! The discrimination and agony this causes is huge. It is a serious life problem for women in many cultures.

Should you wish to read real-life, personal accounts, take a look at the WHO's website, one of many, which sheds light on the plight of women from such communities. In an article called *Mother or nothing: the agony of infertility*, Rita Sembuya, the founder of the Joyce Fertility Support Centre in Uganda, an organisation she set up to support women affected by infertility in Ugandan communities, discusses the difficulties women face.

Sembuya explains that all those who come to her centre for help are universally afflicted by deep anguish and social discrimination. '*Our culture demands that, for a woman to be socially acceptable, she should*

160

have at least one biological child', says Sembuya. *'Almost all cultures across Africa put emphasis on women having children...marriage without children is considered as a failure of the two individuals.".*[17]

To varying degrees and extremes globally, it seems that for many infertility sufferers the struggle to 'fit in', feel included, valued, and even be accepted in communities is a common additional burden. Having a child opens key doors, providing access to otherwise out of bounds social groups, rituals, support and connections, even within families.

Unsurprising that the link between 'reproductive failure' and low self-esteem leading to depression is significant. Most studies establish a direct correlation between infertility and negative self-esteem. Not just in women, also men. Generally though, women with infertility report more 'negative emotions than men, including lower levels of self-esteem and higher levels of depression, anxiety, stigma and shame'.[18]

Further evidence shows that these rock bottom levels of self-esteem can swiftly lead to depression. Not necessarily the other way around though. Researchers Julia Sowislo and Ulrich Orth's study *'Does low self-esteem predict depression and anxiety? A meta-analysis of longitudinal studies'* [19] looks into the relationship between self-esteem and depression vs. depression and self-esteem, if a person has low self-esteem, there's an increased risk of developing depression. This is a very important discovery because it shows that improving a person's self-esteem can make him or her feel better. Depression isn't always linked to low self-esteem. But low-self-esteem can often lead to depression.[20]

Depression is powerful and sly. It's able to suppress, change, and corrode personalities, whilst kept hidden from others and from yourself to a certain degree. Few around me had any inkling what had slithered into my daily life. It wasn't immediately obvious to the casual observer. I wasn't even aware because, being permanently overwhelmed, I couldn't think straight. I felt hopeless, and trapped with that persistent ache in my solar plexus.

I found it difficult to get enthused about activities that I used to be passionate about. I didn't want to go out. My sleep patterns changed. I woke suddenly and couldn't get back to sleep. I was so tired. My focus and concentration were frustratingly blurry. I struggled to multi-task, a skill that's essential in my profession. So, I struggled in some aspects of my job. I had a low tolerance for my own 'mistakes', criticising myself regularly. I couldn't remember details of conversations that I'd only recently had. The list goes on.

To top it off, I'd developed a worrying preoccupation with my malfunctioning womanhood, internalising a lot of frustration with my body. Infertility can have such a destructive influence on our relationships with our bodies. In stark contrast to my procreating peers, not producing a baby had eroded my self-confidence hugely. I felt abnormal. It seemed that every female on the planet on the cusp of motherhood managed it with ease, whilst I was a walking disaster. A fraud! Going through the motions, pretending to be normal. Cruelly let down by my body repeatedly, my body's shortcomings shamed me.

As women, often, consciously or subconsciously, how we function biologically, and the expectations we have of how our bodies should be, look, feel is linked to self-esteem. Hormonally, if nothing else we can't get off the hook. Sure, some of us are fortunate and aren't affected as much as others by a monthly cascade of hormones. I never was. I had no mood swings as such.

As I got older though, and when periods signalled failure, hormones didn't help at all! Casual self-reproach for my defective, inferior femininity became my modus operandi. Why wasn't I biologically like every other woman? Yes, they said there was problem, but we had physical evidence that my husband could father a child, so really it must be me, I reasoned. (It transpired that I too did have a significant issue when it came to regularly ovulating, but this wasn't discovered until later.) After each inexplicable IVF failure, it was my womb that had failed to keep our embryos alive after all.

Upset. Angry. Confused. Paranoid. Anxious. Scared. Isolated. Exhausted. Trying to hide it, and function normally. I needed to feel better and stronger to start the second IVF, but was struggling to get there. I felt a hopeless failure. But didn't want to complain, in case others thought I was making a fuss over a minor issue.

Brit resolve is legendary. The 'just keep going, come what may' mentality. 'Come on! It's not that bad. Just get on with it.' A colleague at work more or less said this to me. Far from being a motivational speech, it had the opposite effect! Culturally, a stiff upper lip approach is entrenched in us Brits when it comes to certain things, especially feelings. Things are improving. Recently, there's been a focus on mental health awareness, and well-being due to some high-profile campaigns.

It's been a sadness and a salve to reflect on how for much of my thirties, I wasn't the woman of my twenties or forties. I feel a little sad about that. For almost a decade, my confidence evaporated, and my personality at home was shrouded by an intermittent dark, heavy cloak. It's sad that the woman my husband had got know, and had helped him, became a kind of someone else. *'I felt a bit of emotional turmoil at that time. I wanted to be able to help my wife more. After all, she had helped me face, overcome and address certain things that I'd not been able to address on my own and hadn't been going that well when we'd first got together, things I'd been struggling with. I wanted to reciprocate.'*

'Like she had helped me to balance things out, to look at my own well-being, to look after myself more, I wanted to give her a sense of calm and reassurance. But whilst she would find the right moment, and talk to me when she saw I needed help, (not in a bossy way, just bringing to the surface areas that needed my attention.) It's not something that comes as naturally to me as it does to her. Sometimes, I felt like I made things worse when I was trying to help her with her emotions. I was out of my depth. I could see her struggling and fading away, but I really didn't know how best to help her. I turned to my mother-in-law a lot at that time for guidance, and advice.'

Having his wife swept away by something that neither of us could fully comprehend or could control was difficult. It ate up so much of his/our time and energies, resources that could've been used for other more fruitful, fulfilling things. But that's depression for you. It's extremely selfish. It doesn't care!

Now, thankfully, I understand. I've finally been able to let go of the embarrassment, and self-admonishment. I no longer listen to those lies that I told myself. That I should be ashamed of my behaviour, for not coping better, for failing. I've been able to apply truth and self-compassion to say, 'Heck, it was tough. There's no shame in that! You did your best with what you had. You acted with integrity and dignity as best you could. Be proud! You did it! You were down, but you rose up again. You came through it. Your marriage survived. You survived. You're a warrior woman!'

Not to overstate the point, but for others in the same boat, it's important to tell it as it was and now is. Now, I give myself permission to acknowledge and respect how I felt. That is the way it was. And now I am a new version of me. Like a phoenix from the flames. Stronger, wiser, a little haggard perhaps, and sometimes still sad, but no longer ashamed or anxious.

'You may write me down in history
With your bitter, twisted lies,
You may trod me in the very dirt
But still, like dust, I'll rise.'[21]

Defeated

P4wM5Crl1a

Here I sit.
I admit defeat.
I'm lifeless, empty.
I'm incomplete.

My hands are up.
I surrender.
I've no more to give.
My heart's too tender.

Too weary to think.
No thought emerges.
Just nothingness,
no drive, no urges.

I'm a desiccated husk
without tears to shed.
I've wept them all.
I'm shrivelled, brittle, dead.

Head on cool stone,
resting hot, sore eyes.
I think of all
we've sacrificed

and what we've lost.
I'm worn out.
Beaten by fear
and hopeless doubt.

My silent pleas,
such foolish prayers!
Desperately said.
But God doesn't care.

Slowly I stand,
start to tremble, shake,
my heavy limbs
throb and ache.

As I take a step,
blame brings a thought,
layering anxieties.
Maybe it is my fault.

Will I ever break this cycle?
Will the day ever dawn
when I'm free from worry,
self-loathing and scorn?

I imagine it.
Relief flooding in
like sudden morning sun
to warm cold as ice skin.

For a fleeting moment
my tension eases,
swept high into the air by a gust
of imagined breezes.

From these dark depths,
will I too rise, soon?
Back into light, freed
from incarcerated gloom.

CHAPTER 18
Faith and fertility

'I prayed for this child, and the Lord has granted me what I asked of
him.'

~

1 Samuel 1:27 (NIV)

Religion isn't everyone's idea of a rollicking read, but globally, political
ideology, cultural traditions and religion are huge influencers regarding
procreation and social stigma. Depending on country or region, each
underpins, to varying degrees, our social outlooks, beliefs, structures,
hierarchy, relationships and identities.

My own upbringing impacted the way I valued myself as a childless
woman later in life. I felt there existed a lot of stigma for childless
married women within the religion I grew up with. Even now in some
progressive religious communities, I would say that there's still a need
for greater representation and a stronger voice for those without
children.

With the exception of Buddhism, family is considered to be at the heart
of most of the world's main religions. In Muslim communities, family and
raising your children well are fundamental values that underpin society.
Inter-religiously and interdenominationally, many teachings and
sermons promote the importance of family, extended family, close
blood relatives, and most critically relationships between parents and
children.

The Church of England views God as the father presiding over his flock of children. The whole set up is structured around this family model, or at the very least this imagery and rhetoric. Thirty years ago, in the three different churches to which I was taken, there was heavy emphasis on the importance of children. This was explicitly taught and felt.

Fertility is at the very heart of the Christian story. Crikey, the whole of the Christian faith is based on heavenly intervention to conceive! I am not a theologian. I won't launch into a protracted theological commentary. But in the context of infertility, my self-esteem as an adult was affected by the religious input I'd had as a child.

Every Sunday, Biblical stories, parables, and teachings were deconstructed, analysed, and retold from various angles and viewpoints. Stories of barren women seemed to be a firm favourite. The plights of women unable, or who struggled to have children, had me waking in cold sweats in adulthood. (Well, not quite, but you get my point!) Stories that had infiltrated my mind as a child were subconsciously influencing my mind many years later.

Infertility, or barrenness, is not usually portrayed in a sympathetic light. Often a source divine punishment, infertility is a key preoccupation in several of the Bible's chapters. In the Old Testament, there's an awful lot of 'womb opening and shutting'[22] being dished out! Please note: all women, no men being struck with this 'curse'!

Even when applying the socio-historical context, these stories can be really disheartening for those in a modern-day similar predicament. 'You will be blessed more than any other people; none of your men or women will be childless...' [23] Message: Children are blessings! 'Behold, children are a heritage from the Lord, the fruit of the womb a reward.'[24]

Message: Children are gifts and rewards from God! Okay. Okay. Enough! Kids are the bee's knees, and if you haven't been 'blessed' with any then consider yourself divinely spurned and castigated! It's a proper telling off. A seat in the naughty corner!

Crisis can strengthen personal faith, draw folk back into the fold, repel them, or reshape entire belief systems. I fell into the latter category, but not without years of talking to, listening for and bargaining with the silent creator-on-a-cloud of my youth. God's apparent indifference added to my bewildered confusion.

Although I wasn't a regular church goer, faith had been on my mind on and off throughout our first three IVF rounds. (By the fourth, I'd modified my strategy.) After the first transfer, entering the precarious stage as guardian of live embryos, I needed quiet time and space. I instinctively made a beeline for a small parish church that happened to be on our route home from the clinic.

Crossing the threshold of a cold, stone, stained glass windowed, wooden-pewed empty chapel sends tingles down my spine. The smaller, least pretentious the better. Perhaps it's something about a church's history. That prayer and suffering, hope and disappointment are as integral to its spiritual architecture as brick and stone are to its physical composition. The Christian Church has had a decidedly chequered past (and present) but for centuries during great hardships, war, disease, famine and poverty these buildings have stood as symbols of hope and refuge in many communities.

So, there I was, sitting alone in a pew at the front of an empty nave, telling a distant, silent God about our embryos, tears rolling down my cheeks. I asked that they would be kept alive. I asked to be released from such a draining cycle.

Needless to say, hope and prayer were obliterated by disillusionment and despair in the wake of each loss. Yet again, my husband bore the brunt of pacifying my anguished outbursts. 'What have I done to deserve this? Why is this happening to me? It's not fair! Don't I deserve my own child?' A diatribe that under normal circumstances was out of character. When it comes to grief, like depression, personality and outlook can be distorted entirely! Rationally, I knew life doesn't dish out just deserts in some kind of weird ranking system! Terrible, unjust things happen to innocent and blameless people all the time. To people who don't 'deserve' it.

The second half of this reproach took place internally, along the lines of, 'What gives you the right to complain about such a trivial matter? Many have greater traumas to face. Terminal cancer, neurodegenerative diseases, life changing illnesses, fatal accidents, losing loved ones, war, natural disasters... Dreadful human suffering is happening across the globe. And here you are, whining about infertility! The world is overpopulated. Not producing more humans is a good thing for the planet! Get over it! Ridiculous! God doesn't even exist! You're wasting your breath'. This self-talk could go one of two ways; helping to keep perspective, or heaping on more guilty negativity for acting churlish and entitled!

Faith and fertility – a big subject. Such a personal journey. I never totally lost hope in a miracle. (I think until it's finally curtains for me reproductively speaking, and the menopause comes along, I will continue to be teased by that desperate flicker of 'just maybe this time'.)

My faith in some ways added further sadness and disappointment rather than being a consistent source of strength.

Since then, I've had to work at getting my faith to where it is now. Reconfiguring it into something that brings more freedom. More peace and positivity. No anxiety. More self-acceptance and less self-reproach. I've found great solace and sanctuary in my quiet morning reflections, meditations, and runs on my own in the outdoors. I have renewed optimism in my remodelled concept of connection to self and to one another. This has evolved after much soul searching, listening and learning, sharing and talking.

Perhaps I wouldn't have struggled with my faith so much had I already been a part of an established supportive, pro-feminist, faith community when all of this was taking place. Maybe I would've had more light when I was walking in those long shadows. As the wise cleric, and human rights activist Sir Desmond Tutu says, finding light, finding our gateway to hope for something better, is paramount to maintaining mental balance and our overall well-being.

I'm slightly envious of those whose faith is a more consistent source of encouragement and reassurance. It's intriguingly admirable. I often thought of Terry Waite, the hostage negotiator kidnapped in Lebanon in 1987. A powerful source of inspiration when I was young, his book, *Taken on Trust* is a must read for all those with an interest in human endurance, inner strength, resilience, humility, and of course, hope and faith. His remarkable example grounded me in difficult moments. '...*if you have faith, you will not be destroyed, and you will find that you can live in hope.*'[25] His story helped me understand the true meaning of resilience, courage and strength.

My sister-in-law, who has had her wobbles through her own fertility journey, has remained steadfast in her faith. In moments of doubt and anguish, her faith has been an integral part of her support structure throughout trying to conceive. It has been comforting to know that she and my brother belong to a supportive community that's responsive to their needs as a couple who've experienced failed IVF.

Whilst others might be cynical of faith-based practices, I'm thankful for the community that this can offer. In our case, as we are in Spain and they're in the UK, and especially as they're actively involved in helping their wider local community, I'm grateful for those who lifted them up and stood by them. I asked my sister-in-law for her thoughts on the subject.

'My church friends have been supportive. I have a WhatsApp group of a few girlfriends and whenever I'm feeling low, I message them and they send messages of encouragement. When my first IVF failed, these ladies checked in regularly, came round for coffee, and dropped round flowers and cards. The main issue for me in our church community is that 99% of my friends have young children. I find christenings difficult. I want to celebrate the babies, and I enjoy spending time with my friend's children, but it makes my heart (and ovaries) ache for my own.'

'I put pressure on myself to be a mother to share that experience with my friends. It was something I've wanted since senior school. I've always felt as if I had to catch up with them as they all got married when I was single; then I got married, they started to have children whilst I struggled to conceive.'

'There doesn't seem to be a balance between those with children and those without. There are lots of families that have children, and only a

few that don't. Generally though, my church is inclusive and encouraging of women without children. I've found attending inspirational women-only gatherings very uplifting. Having said that, many events are very family orientated – picnics or family days which is difficult. I don't feel comfortable going along just as a couple without children.'

'There are a group of church mums, friends of mine, who meet at a local café most Friday mornings for coffee and a catch up with their children. I joined them once, but it was difficult. My friends didn't intentionally make it hard, but there was much of the conversation that I couldn't contribute to as they were discussing their kids.'

'Within our church community, I've felt supported and encouraged through the IVF process and haven't been afraid to ask for support. If I was to give advice to any faith-based community, then it would be to BE INCLUSIVE. Don't favour women with children over those who are childless. Also, please don't expect a childless woman to give more time just because she doesn't have children so will have 'more time'!'

'Trying to conceive has definitely challenged my beliefs. I´ve been through different stages depending on my mood (and time of the month!) which is good as authenticity and being real is important. I've had dark moments when I've felt totally abandoned, and I have shouted out asking why we haven't been able to get pregnant when we are both so desperate to become parents. Then on good days, I remember to trust that the right people will be put in our path to encourage and empower us to keep us going.' Heidi

God, are you listening?

God, are you listening?
I'm worn out from my grief.
My eyes are sore and swollen.
I cannot find relief.

God, why aren't you listening?
Many nights tears drench my bed.
A continual ache is throbbing
throughout my body and in my head.

God, have you forgotten me?
Why do you hide when I need you most?
My soul, like sand, is scattered by the wind.
Though my heart beats, I'm but a ghost.

God, have you forsaken me?
Why do you feel so far away?
I need refreshment and encouragement.
My strength is dried up like sun-baked clay.

God, can you hear me?
Each night I cry out for your help.
I thought that you might rescue me.
I feel so alone and by myself.

God, why do you ignore my pleas?
I'm out of depth in this deep water.
I'm no match for this mighty sea.
Be a rock for me, your humble daughter.

God, do you even exist?
Answer me, for sanity's sake.
My faith is all but vanished though I see you
in mighty mountains, and misted lake.

God, can you please be merciful?
For I am in great distress.
You say that you will watch over me
in times of fear and great sadness.

God, have you rejected me?
I am shrivelled, waiting for your blessing.
I wish to be like a captive bird,
released from her cage, so utterly depressing.

God, are you punishing me?
Is there something wrong that I have done?
Send your light, and your truth,
let me not by my thoughts be undone.

God, will I find peace one day?
Where does my shadowy path lead me?
Don't abandon me in my hour of need,
walk beside me on my journey.

God, will you rescue me?
Clinging hopeless to this barren life.
I wish to be like a thriving olive tree,
fruitful, beautiful, blossoming, alive.

God, do you remember me?
Have you been with me since birth?
Did you see me in my mother's womb?
A future of integrity, positivity and worth.

O silent God, why don't you listen?
My plea is founded in fragile, humility.
Though I try to be a valiant, warrior woman,
I need help conquering this curse of infertility.

CHAPTER 19

Talk to me

'You have to be able to talk about your mental health, in order to be mentally fit and therefore, be happy, healthy, for the rest of your life. You have to talk about your mental fitness.'

~

Prince Harry

Out of darkness comes light! Isn't it amazing when we have that lightbulb moment? For me, this usually happens when I've given myself time and space to think clearly, read, write, listen to a good podcast, or talk with a friend who 'gets it' – who understands how to help my 'mental fitness.' On this occasion though, a splendid bolt of enlightenment struck during a relationship counselling session. Counselling was what really turned the tide.

There had been a specific, very precarious, crisis moment after which I'd instructed my husband to source the best relationship psychotherapist he could find locally, and book us both in as soon as possible. For 6 months, we went regularly. The aim was to understand each other better, to rediscover a healthy, enjoyable life together, and to deal with and heal from all of the crappiness that had been flung at us over the years. In short, to save our relationship and our sanity!

During one of the sessions, we were given a handout called 'The Rollercoaster of Loss'. For me, the penny kerplunked. 'So there is an acknowledged, perfectly normal pattern for grief! Maybe I wasn't such a loon, after all!' The ensuing discussion focused on the 5 or 7 stages of loss.[26] 'Wow! This is me!' I marvelled.

Each stage represented my journey quite clearly. **Shock** – and confusion that we were having problems conceiving. **Denial** – not believing it. Still waiting for a baby to materialise. **Anger** – at the injustice and unfairness of our situation. **Bargaining** – and pleading with a higher 'power', making unrealistic deals with myself. **Depression** – feeling utterly hopeless, lost and sad. **Testing** – feeling calmer, more positive moments, able to think more clearly. **Acceptance** – acknowledging that there is a positive way forward. Talking about and understanding this, I began to let go and trust this process rather than berate myself for it.

My second cerebral spark came a few months later, when I enrolled on a college course. Needing new direction, and motivation, I began studying for a Counselling Skills qualification. Anyone who has juggled family life with work and extra study will understand my pride in this. I was teaching part time by then, attending college a day a week, completing weekly reading and written assignments.

What a breath of fresh air, and how invaluable the skills and knowledge have since been! Developing self-awareness and having a better grasp on what makes us tick as humans still has fantastically tangible benefits to my personal and professional life. I use these 'life skills' in every area. It's great that something so positive came from a place that had felt so hopeless.

Have you ever experienced this? How, when you look back some time later, at a moment of bleakness when all had seemed lost, and you've come out the other side, there is goodness that has subsequently taken root and grown from it? This has happened to me various times.

As for my angry outbursts, it was liberating to know that they were a normal, healthy part of the grieving process. I wasn't a failure or bad person. It was inevitable that I would feel this way. If only I'd realised this sooner, it could've saved years of pointless self-flagellation! Anger is, for short periods, necessary. (Not in an out-of-control smashing plates, totally loco, dangerous way, obviously!) It would've been healthier if, I'd understood that strong emotions are a natural and necessary part of healing. Grief must be released if we're to move on to a more peaceful place.

Why didn't I go back to my GP, clinic, or get robust professional help sooner? So much could've been avoided had we had proper immediate support. I suppose that though it seems glaringly obvious now, like the frog, sometimes you aren't aware of how bad it's become. Perhaps it takes someone else to point it out and say, 'It *is* ok not to be ok, but you need help to get back to being ok!' Instead of covering it up all the time, it's a darned relief when you do finally take that leap of faith to talk about what's been eating away at you, which is exactly what my husband's friend had done all those years ago when he suggested my husband seek mental health help after the birth of his daughter.

Recently, I asked him why he'd recommended psychotherapy to my husband back then, why he thought it could help, '*It had helped me. When I was just starting my career I suffered from a lot of work stress which was seriously affecting my mental health, and my doctor recommended psychotherapy. I was doubtful, but it totally rocked my world, like a secret shortcut back to feeling normal.*'

'*Ever since then I've guarded my mental health as my most valuable possession. I don't understand why people acknowledge that they need a professional to help with plumbing, for example, but won't hire someone to help them deal with psychological issues.'* So, if you need help, and haven't tried psychotherapy, do. Go for it! It could totally *'rock your world'* too.

To say I didn't have any helpful professional counselling to prepare me for IVF, wouldn't be entirely true. I'd had regular reflexology with a lady called Liz, an amazingly kind, expert reflexologist. She was by chance, also a trained metaphysical counsellor. So, a serendipitous by-product was that whilst my feet were receiving care, my mind had valuable TLC too.

I learnt from her wise self-care advice. And I wasn't the only one who benefitted. Once, when my husband came to collect me, Liz glided out of the house, gracefully down the drive, and gently, but firmly informed my husband through the car window that he too needed to be kinder to himself and find more balance in his demanding life. He nodded meekly, agreeing to make more effort. Ah, Liz. I couldn't help, but chuckle.

There was also of course, my remarkable mother without whom we'd have certainly crumbled. The unwavering insightful counsel that this patient woman provided was priceless. She should be canonised, or receive an MBE for services to mental health at the very least! No matter what, she was always ready to listen, talk, and encourage. She's a prevailing source of light and inspiration for many, not just us. We always felt comfortable and safe talking with her. Never judged, threatened or wasting her time. Many could learn a lot from her attitude to helping others. She should do a TED talk!

Putting someone at ease, ensuring a person feels comfortable before you start any therapy or intervention is super important. Who the heck is going to feel ready to divulge difficult details of their life if the environment is unsuitable, the conditions are counterintuitive, or the counsellor's own communication is out of whack? Adult or child, we know we're being truly authentically listened to. Then we feel seen, and fully valued.

It's rare to listen without seeking to impart our own agendas and opinions. Without interrupting, butting in, chipping in with our own anecdotes. Listening isn't about us and our own egos. It's about caring for the other person. Being truly heard, acknowledges who we are. We feel appreciated, understood. Each of us needs this validation. Feeling valued boosts our self-esteem and sense of self-worth.

Non-verbal communication is extremely powerful, more so than verbal. Did you know that most experts agree that only 7% of communication is verbal, meaning that approximately 93% is non-verbal? We listen with our whole body through posture, facial expressions, gestures, movements.[27] If we're nodding without looking up from our phones, or not putting them to one side to give our whole attention, what is this communicating? We listen with our eyes as much as our ears. We are saying, 'I see you. I've got you.' Candid, healing conversations can then take place as we feel held, safe and valued.

Unfortunately, not all trained professionals manage this approach. Our first IVF counsellor, for example, as wet as a fish with a handshake as limp as a noodle, looked as if she were in pain, and could do with seeing a therapist herself! She didn't inspire confidence. The session was astonishingly awkward. We couldn't get out of there fast enough.

Our second counsellor's use of long, aloof silences (intended, we supposed, to encourage us to talk) and habit of staring off into the middle distance over our shoulders was also most off-putting. We fared no better with her! These were both counsellors provided by the clinic as a one-off part of our original package.

So, how can fertility clinics and hospitals get the basics of the counselling experience right? For starters, I would emphatically advise paying attention to the details, i.e., room, surroundings, chairs, décor, location, heating! etc. In short, providing comfort and safety in a pleasant, appropriate environment with professionals who are at the top of their game. The couple have just lost their future children. For crying out loud, put a pot plant in the corner! Invest in comfortable chairs at the very least! An unwelcoming, clinical, chilly corner of a medical facility is hardly the place for sensitive discussions about trauma and loss. The austere, bare hospital room that doubled as our counselling area the first time was enough to bring on paper-bag breathing just from entering the room.

But that was a blast compared to a dear friend of mine's experience. She was living a waking nightmare. Her first baby, after a full term, healthy pregnancy, had inexplicably died in her womb just days before her due date. My friend gave birth to her daughter, Gloria - tragically stillborn. It's almost impossible to comprehend the sheer scale of this horror. Instead of a new-born in her arms, she left hospital carrying an agony too traumatic and all-consuming to even begin to describe. Unimaginable pain. How do you resume life in the face of such tragedy? You definitely need professional help and care. Grief counselling was offered which she took.

Imagine then, plucking up the courage to return to the same hospital to talk to your recommended counsellor. Imagine the long walk down the same corridor, through the same antenatal ward packed with pregnant mums and new mothers with babies where my friend had been only weeks before to give birth. Imagine the relief upon finding the counselling room door on that ward, knocking, and waiting to be ushered in. Imagine your knock unanswered, turning to sit in the waiting area, those minutes ticking by to the cries of new-borns, and murmurs of mothers - your own body alive with hormones, physically yearning for your own child. Your loss is suffocating you, but you've no choice but to wait. Imagine the self-control not to run screaming back down the corridor.

Then, imagine if you will, your barely-out-of-her-teens counsellor arriving cheerily clutching a Styrofoam coffee, breezily apologising for 'running a bit late' casually unlocking the door. 'She had time to pick up that damn coffee!' My friend, my dear incredible friend. Another true warrior woman! Needless to say, she never went back, opting instead for a private specialist with an altogether different approach.

I was incredulous and incensed when told this. It backed up my theory at the lack of adequate care for women and couples with fertility related loss. Obviously, losing a child in this way is different to failed fertility treatment, but it's linked. There are troubling shortcomings in effective psychological care for patients. It seems that in both public and private sectors, the lack of robust and meaningful care is alarmingly commonplace.

In the previously mentioned *Fertility Network UK Survey on the Impact of Fertility Problems*, shockingly, 56% of respondents didn't have any counselling after failed IVF treatment. And of the small group that did, a quarter describe it as 'a ticking boxes exercise' only. One of several recommendations given in this report was for substantial improvements to be made, '*Funded counselling is needed at appropriate times and with an appropriate focus, including supporting people with unsuccessful treatment outcomes or relationship difficulties'.*[28]

This report is not unique in its findings. Evidence indicating that more adequate support is needed can be found from a variety of sources. Yet although the psychological impact is widely recognised and understood by fertility specialists, it remains an area that's worryingly overlooked and neglected.

US psychologist, Dr Allyson Bradow, in her study of the psychological effects of fertility treatments, states that some patients risk developing Post Traumatic Stress Disorder after multiple failed treatments. Farfetched? In her study, almost 50 percent of fertility patient participants met the PTSD official criteria. This ties in with a further focus of the *Fertility Network UK* report regarding the high levels of distress and trauma infertility sufferers experience.

Whilst I don't recommend self-diagnosis of serious medical conditions, I am partial to an online quiz when the mood takes me! Ten minutes and a few clicks later, hey presto, I'd pretty much diagnosed myself with PTSD! Clearly, if you are concerned about yourself or a family member, seeking expert help as soon as possible is advisable. For me, the test was more a retrospective experiment.

Considering the cost of private treatment, these findings add to the audacious lack of appropriate care. Do some clinics just take the money and run as various media reports suggest? Despite spending thousands, when we were asked in our follow up consultations if we wanted further IVF cycles, once we'd said that we needed to think and reconfigure financially, we never heard from any of our clinics again! No routine check back from our consultant or nurses on either our physical or mental well-being. Nothing to help with emotional management apart from of course, the strangely awkward tick-box counselling. Like many couples, we were left entirely alone to fend for ourselves.

Let's talk

rPCaudmCz8

Let's talk
Dig out muddled thoughts
and talk to me
Let's talk
about your feelings patiently
I'll listen
wait until you find your flow
I'll listen
tension on your face
you're feelin' low
I see you need care
I'll take care with you
I see you've lost hope
I'll guide you through
Trust your unconscious mind
Let go and you will find
emotions bring words

I understand
relax more if you can
Let's talk
Let's talk
Let's talk, be honest
about your fears
Let's talk, reflect
your mind'll clear
I'll listen with gentle wisdom
I'll listen. I'm used to problems
Real serious problems
I'll respect what you say
with empathy
You're weighed down by pain
and anxiety
In this safe and peaceful space
just go at your own pace
Take your time, it's really tough
little wonder you've had enough!

CHAPTER 20
Self-care or self-combust!

'The only way we can begin to see more clearly, and see another way, is to give ourselves space. It might only be five minutes before beginning our workday ... and yes, every one of us can find five minutes if we want to.'

~

Sháá Wasmund

It doesn't make us ungrateful narcissists when what's dumped on our doorsteps overwhelms us. We may not be escaping war zones, living in famine and disease ravaged countries, or refugee camps, but our experiences are still valid and relevant. It's natural for things in our own lives to be stressful and painful. Infertility sucks. And it's ok to say so.

Through honest, empowering conversations with two fantastic therapists (at different times) I learnt to be honest and stop fighting myself. To feel better, we must give ourselves permission to feel sad, to cry, to ask for help, to understand our feelings, and to grieve our failed treatments, our 'lost' embryos, and unresolved childlessness. We shouldn't feel guilty or ashamed!

Being kind to ourselves, practising self-compassion, and being aware of our emotional stamina levels are key to survival. We must be realistic with what we can and cannot manage. This varies from person to person of course. Even though we know this, it's easy to fall into the trap of comparing ourselves with others, feeling we should be more like them. But in reality, we've no idea what is being concealed behind closed doors. Everyone operates differently, has different strengths and challenges.

To rediscover our own 'personal peace' and confidence we must first understand who we are, and work with what we've got, rather than preoccupying ourselves with who we think we ought to be, and what we think we ought to have! This requires self-awareness and courage. The more aware and accepting we are of ourselves, the less likely we are to be sucked into that spiralling vortex of insecurities and self-doubt. The more courageous we become, the more we can stand firm to be ourselves without fearing reprisal through the words and attitudes of others.

As I increasingly understood these two key, life-changing 'philosophies', the kinder, more self-compassionate I became, more able to monitor and take responsibility for my stamina levels. Instead of allowing myself to be dragged repeatedly beyond suitable parameters, I became a more congruous decision maker. I guess this could also be called wisdom and balance. My expectations changed and goal posts moved to be more in line with the realities of my own life, needs, personality and relationships. And the more determined, less fearful I became about doing this.

Life for parents of young children is child-centred, and, depending on their age, often all-consuming. They need help with most things day and night. Much of our emotional, physical and mental selves are invested in childcare and child-rearing. When my stepdaughter was small, sometimes she woke with night terrors. My husband or I would cradle her back to sleep. When shampoo stung her eyes at bath-time, I put on silly voices to make her laugh! I transformed cereal boxes into Barbie's shower, made treasure hunts, prepared picnics, and organised holiday projects. I would help her perform song and dance routines for Daddy. And when tantrums got the better of her, we would wait until tearful and red-faced, she said sorry, climbing onto our laps for cuddles. With her, our home was a wonderful hive of activity, family and energy. Without her, our home felt empty. Dolls and crayons, bikes and swimming paraphernalia were packed away again.

On one hand, the return to our childfree existence bought relative peace, tranquillity and, a wonderfully uncluttered home! On the other, her absence re-activated the ache. The contrast of life with my stepdaughter, and our ordinarily quiet home was disorientatingly conspicuous. I used to give everything I had in my emotional cache to her visits, leaving nothing left to cope with the fall out of giving her up again. Adapting and acclimatising each time through this strange hinterland was exhausting, completely sapping our emotional stamina levels.

However, once we acknowledged and planned for this, the easier transitions became. The kinder we were to ourselves. We looked after each other more. Although, it didn't come naturally and still doesn't to my husband, we had more realistic expectations of what we should permit on our personal life plates, especially during, and just after those transitions. Slowly, we were learning the art of self-care and well-being.

Preserving our sanity, adapting to life with infertility, when many of our buddies are busy preserving theirs adapting to life as new parents, takes thought and effort. Whilst new parent posses are sprouting up left, right and centre, infertility sufferers join the...well...there's not really an obvious gang, unless you go out of your way to find one! I advise making concerted efforts to cultivate our own alternative tribes, broadening who we spend time with, not in a divisive way, but in a balanced, self-compassionate way.

Seeking out, and investing in friendships that will nurture us, reignite our sparks, and fill up our tanks rather than depleting them, is a very good thing! What are our hobbies? What do we enjoy doing with other like-minded people? I get a natural high from singing, so I joined a soul choir to help keep me topped up with positive creativity. What a buzz! It was brilliant to connect with new people in safety, away from children. This did my confidence, and mental space the world of good.

This may sound controversial. I'm not suggesting ditching our friends because they suddenly have kids. I'm merely highlighting the need for healthy, realistic, balanced input. When we're having a difficult week fertility-wise, why would we choose to spend our free, emotional down time with those with babies? Of course, sometimes it's unavoidable, but generally, should we put ourselves in that situation if we're already struggling?

As I've said, before I knew better, I did just that. I should've prioritised more time with friends who were able to provide a safe environment, non-child related conversational content, and a calm mental haven - imperative for those who find themselves developing anxiety issues when it comes to social events, or even leaving the house.

Self-care should be taught in schools as a regular, solid part of everyone's routine. It's not just for those of us who are having a particularly tough time. Setting aside time and space for it should be a priority. We can all do to it if we try. And once we've implemented effective coping strategies, it's vital to be pro-active about sustaining them. It takes trial and error to hone what realistically works for us.

For me, in challenging periods, a combination of talking therapy, increased rest, running (Goodness! I love the endorphin hit from running. Mentally, running has been a very healing and worthwhile practice), writing, cooking and music have been what I needed. We each have our own unique self-care recipe for what works in our busy lives, especially combining it with work pressures too. When work is super busy, it is hard to maintain it. But then, maybe it's time to think out of the box, and get creative.

I asked some friends, fellow fertility challenged ladies what helped them to stay on an even keel particularly when work was demanding too. One friend found that a change of working hours was required. For others, it's a question of positive mental attitude, establishing healthier boundaries, and learning to say no to what we know will tip us over the edge. Here's what some had to say.

'Be kind to yourself and don't force yourself to be in situations that may be too difficult or will have negative ramifications. I found being open with people was the best strategy, usually resulting in greater understanding and kindness. Find a fertility practitioner you can trust and have faith in. Adjust your expectations of yourself, so that they're kinder, more realistic. It's your journey and only you can decide how that is to be travelled.' Sarah

'I actually found a great deal of comfort in the fact that I could carry on doing my job through it all. It really helped me to remind myself that though I might be a royal disaster in the reproductive arena, I was still a valuable member of society! My value to those around me was far greater than the functioning (or lack thereof) of my uterus and fallopian tubes! I found that if we act brave, we become brave. This was my experience. So soldier on! Also, it helped a great deal to rest after work.

It made my work life a lot easier. I would go home and nap every day with a little meditation thrown in.' Karen

'I was concerned about my mental health. I was fortunate as I was able to change my contract to part time, working three days a week. If you are unhappy at work, then look for solutions to make it better. If changing or quitting your job feels like the right thing to do, then do it. Do not dwell on it. It really did help. Learning to say no to taking on too much work, going for walks at lunchtime, reducing my working hours and workload helped me feel less stressed. The more you can do to make your life less busy and stressful, the better.' Dina

'Take each day at a time. Be kind to yourself – if you are having a bad day and feel sad, allow yourself to feel the pain – don't have a pity party – but allow yourself a set amount of time to grieve. When there is no way to avoid a situation with a pregnant woman or families, think through how you will react and then give yourself time to decompress afterwards. I also need time alone to chill and sort things out in my head. I like playing on the games console – nothing too mentally taxing! Part of my self-care has been to see a counsellor regularly to talk about what is bothering me and being challenged about the way I think about things. I believe in the power of words and that saying positive words to yourself can affect your mood and how you react to things. Finally, take each day at a time. If that is too hard, just take each hour at a time.' Heidi

'It was definitely the hardest thing I've ever been through. There were days when I wanted to stay curled up on the sofa and cry all day. There were others when I suffered from anxiety and making decisions. Going out just seemed too hard. Personal mantras and positive visualisation made things easier. Just be kind to yourself. Treat yourself with love and kindness. Put that self-care above all else. If you do need to have a day

at home on the sofa, take it and don't feel guilty. Your sanity is more important. Daily meditation, the visualisation and mantras helped me considerably, but you also need to surround yourself with lovely people. You need a support crew. Let the people who say the offensive things drift out of your circle for the time being.' Ruth

Such good advice! Not a one size fits all approach. How we're able to practice self-care will differ, although the fundamentals remain the same. The message is clear. We should be self-compassionate! I urge you to find what works best for you. Ruth is so right when she mentions a support crew as we adapt and make these choices and changes. If some people we care about aren't able to say or do the right thing, take a little breather from them. And if we can't, we should balance them out with those whom we trust to always have our backs and make us feel good, spending more time with these people, and less with the others.

In fact, this is now one of my general life rules, not just regarding infertility. Identify those who don't drain us, and spend time with them. Nurture friendships with people who do not reprimand us, or belittle our loss when we feel sad. Prioritise time with those who instead of bringing us down, we trust to listen, lift us up, encourage, and champion us.

Problems

c6M2UIUgTQ

Why are you writing this stuff down?
You should be enjoying life. You're in your prime!
If you want real problems to write about,
I can give you some of mine.

Let me tell you about troubles, girl.
You don't know nothing about the daily grind.
Waking up every morning
with a hundred problems on your mind.

'Normal' people just get on with it.
When asked, they say, 'I'm fine.'
Behind closed doors they deal with it
with a bottle of cheap red wine.

Where's your Brit resolve, stiff upper lip?
Your determination and grit?
You ain't going to win no battles with poetry,
where's your fighting spirit?

Anyway, who has time to write,
rest, do yoga, walk, hug a leafy tree?
I battle on without these antics,
and I'm fine, just look at me.

Meditation's overrated, a gimmick.
Counselling, well that's a joke.
Just quacks who charge you megabucks
to meddle in the private lives of 'normal' folk.

You're focusing too much on negativity.
Grumbles, whinging and whines.
I'm sure that you'd perk right up,
if you didn't bang on about problems all the time.

Who's going to read your anecdotes?
We've got enough worries on our plate!
A pandemic, plastic waste, the Brexit mess...
not to mention the rise of a fascist, right wing state.

I've read your poems, they're ok.
Some of them even rhyme.
But you should write some proper gags,
ones with actual funny punchlines!

Writing about issues won't solve them.
We've all got mountains to climb.
Spouting verse like a Shakespearean bard?
What a pointless waste of time.

CHAPTER 21
Fab friends and kinetic kindness

Oh, I get by with a little help from my friends
I get high with a little help from my friends
Gonna try with a little help from my friends

~

The Beatles

True friendship is great, isn't it? Friends who say the right things and make us feel fantastic are so nourishing. 'Soul friends' ignite a light inside us that continues to dance and shine long after our interactions with them. They bring out the best in us, topping up our mojo and reminding us that we are enough, and do have enough resilience to jump our hurdles with integrity and compassion for others.

Strong friendships, that is, meaningful connections provide important well-being benefits. They can even literally help us survive! Yes, we may have to shell out for expert help, we may even need medication to get us through. (No shame in that. Much to my surprise, I've been there.) We may have brilliant relationships with our partners, families, colleagues, pets, but it's not enough. Not, according to science! If we really wish to combat anxiety, boost health, lead happier lives, and live longer, science shows that we should regularly hang out with the right good friends.

Nurturing close, healthy friendships is essential for our psychological health, and our physical health. Remarkably, a 2006 oncology study of nearly 3,000 nurses with breast cancer found that those with 10 or more good friends were four times less likely to die from the disease than those without close friendships. The quality and frequency of contact with those friends wasn't linked to the women's survival rates. It seemed that just by having meaningful, supportive relationships was enough. Later research that took data from 148 studies involving over 300,000 participants, found that in the absence of strong friendships the overall risk of premature death increased by 50%. This risk factor is comparable to smoking up to 15 cigarettes a day, and represents a greater mortality rate than obesity and physical inactivity. Friendship saves lives! Word!

An article by the website Upworthy entitled, 'Women do better when they have a group of strong female friends, study finds'[29] once popped up on my newsfeed. It discussed how a study published in the Harvard Business Review shows that a strong inner circle of female friends can help us thrive in our professional lives too. The study found a correlation between women in higher leadership positions and better pay with having a close-knit group of friends. Our female friends empower us and help us thrive in many aspects of life! So, if we haven't done so for a while, let's pick up the phone, give our buddies a call or message, reconnect with them, remind them they're fabulous, and tell them why we're thankful for their friendship.

We need friendship. Without it, when life's challenges strike, we risk becoming isolated, stressed and overly introspective. A good friend acts as a counterbalance to reassure us, boost morale and build self-esteem. When a friend talks with us, listens and empathises, this replenishes our spiritual, emotional and mental health. Friends are great stress relievers. Quality time with them gives us an oxytocin boost that combats stress hormones such as cortisol, thereby reducing the risk of harmful disease and illness. Scientists say so! Laughter too is great medicine, releasing endorphins – happy hormones. Laughing with our friends improves our mood and helps to pull us out of a funk if we're in one.

The key survival strategy here isn't the more friends the better. The trick is to have a close circle of trustworthy, authentic friends on whom you can rely. It's quality over quantity! A peloton of sisterhood that you don't have to see or communicate with every day. Often, it's enough just to know that they're there. So, let's nurture these friendships and not take them for granted. Let's choose wisely who we invite into our inner circle. And let's remember, a friend is not someone who, when our chips are down and need support, adds to our emotional load, and vice versa.

Just as we would respond to a friend in need, a good friend makes us feel better rather than worse. If that's not happening, then that's not true friendship! The handful of people who we turn to in times of adversity, hardship, and grieving must be those who show compassion and kindness with actions and words. To this end, it's important to be wisely selective about who we confide in and surround ourselves with.

We shouldn't just look outwardly, expecting others to always boost us. We must make sure that we're also responding to our friends. Reciprocity should be balanced so the benefits work both ways. Proactive kindness produces a rather wonderful surge in our dopamine and serotonin levels, changing our brain chemistry, helping us feel more positive and happier even.

As author David R. Hamilton articulates in his book, *The Five Side Effects of Kindness*, focusing outwards, practising compassion and kindness is a powerful tool for those suffering from depression and anxiety. He says, *'Just as focusing on helping others helps alleviate depression, having compassion for the suffering of others takes us out of our own suffering. It stops us focusing on the problems that are causing us worry and stress. It aligns us with our deepest nature. It lets us glimpse a grander part of ourselves, that portion that genuinely wants to see our friends and loved ones happy, and that is happy itself.'* [30]

I love this! Having an attitude of kindness is marvellously healing. If we're open to making kindness a conscious life practice, our whole well-being will benefit. Yes, it takes a little effort when we feel absolutely rubbish. When we're extremely low, it's hard to think straight, let alone switch from an inward focus to an outward expression of loving-kindness, but if we can find the motivation, oh boy, there is abundant healthy goodness in acting this way.

Being kind to others is another way to practice the art of self-compassion, too. By caring for others, I am caring for myself. We're all connected. The Butterfly Effect - the positive ripples that we create - has the potential to reach far beyond our own concerns and lives. I find this a truly powerful concept.

This is how our friends can realistically and appropriately assist. By responding to friends and family members suffering from infertility with love and kindness. Rather than suggesting further fertility techniques, miracle remedies, adoption or offering anecdotal, supposed-to-be-motivational advice or stories, or never even mentioning it, the most wonderful thing I've found that a friend can say is, 'I'm here for you. I'm so sorry this utterly sucks'.

One of the most wonderful things a friend can do is set aside time for us from their busy life. When they know we've really hit a rough patch, a friend who offers to put their kids to bed early, and then cook a meal for the two of you, or order a takeaway so you can spend quality time together gives us a beautifully warm glow. When a friend who is already up to their own eyeballs in their own day-to-day shenanigans, prioritises time with us, and shows us kindness in doing so, wow, it's a hugely empowering boost! One that I'm sure adds at least a couple of years to our life span!

Small gestures make a big difference too. I love my sister-in-law Heidi's friends' response, and her work colleagues' too, to her failed IVF. Each sent her a bouquet of flowers. How thoughtful! When people are kind, it's such a lovely, healing feeling! When our final IVF failed, in a kind of 'pay it forward-esque' way, we received a beautiful surprise bouquet from my sister-in law and brother. In our heartbreak, looking at the gorgeous flowers was a reminder that we weren't alone, that someone was thinking of us in our loss.

Obviously, how we're able to respond to our friends and family in need will differ, but showing our friends love and kindness even in the simplest terms is by far the best strategy to help them overcome and 'survive', particularly grief and loss. I personally attest to this. My own personal challenge: balancing the invisible grief of infertility with the destabilising nature of stepmotherhood, has been made more bearable when my friends have walked beside me with compassion, love and care. This has boosted my morale, put a spring in my step and cheered my soul. It also relieved some of the pressure on my relationship with my husband, benefitting his emotional well-being too.

In fact, right now on my writing desk next to me, sits a small jar that when switched on, lights up. A dozen little star shaped lights in its interior, illuminate the words, 'You can totally do this.' It was given to me by a good friend just before my fourth and final IVF. I'd spoken to her about my deep fear that it wouldn't work, and how it scared me. Together, we shared details of our lives that at that moment we found overwhelming, scary and incredibly testing.

We both gained great strength and courage from that conversation which is now visibly and tangibly represented in the form of the little light up jar. She has one also. As twee as it may sound, it's given me comfort numerous times, especially during this writing process when I've felt like downing tools, slinking off and giving up. Knowing that she has the matching pair, despite our distance as she lives in the UK, we are still connected by our friendship represented by this symbolic gift.

A further uplifting kindness that gives me a warm, empowering glow when I think of it; a celebration dinner that, Vanessa, my friend who'd lost her baby daughter a few years prior, instructed me to book for her and me. I rarely discuss the nitty-gritty of my stepmother challenges with anyone apart from my husband and my mother. But there was a particularly upsetting incident that I was wrestling to overcome. I talked it through on the phone with her. It so happened that she was due to fly out to stay with me a few weeks later.

'Right, lady,' she decreed, 'you're going to book us a special celebration meal. My shout. Research somewhere special. Somewhere really nice where you wouldn't ordinarily go. We'll put on our glad rags and go out to celebrate just how awesome we both are. Because we deserve it. We're amazing. And you are an incredible stepmother. We're going to acknowledge it and celebrate it as my treat to the both of us. Remember, somewhere really special!' So, I did. I booked the most beautiful restaurant in town where, dolled up in our finery, we ate a splendid and expensive meal, toasted each other's fabulousness and just generally enjoyed this wonderful moment of celebrating our friendship thanks to my friend's kind generosity.

Be kind

a9YUdKkn9z

What if there was a little pill
that stopped us getting really ill?
A potion to reduce heart disease.
A recipe for beautiful unclogged arteries.
I'd quaff it down. I'd neck a few shots
to protect myself from rogue blood clots.
Strokes, diabetes, premature arthritis,
the remedy, they say, is simple. It's kindness.
A powerful injection? A healthy feel-good jab?
No. Being kind can't be mixed in a chemist's secret lab!
Altruistic acts slow ageing, help to keep us fit,
regenerate our muscles, lift a downcast spirit.
Healing through acts of compassion.
All it takes is outward expression
of kindness. Real human connection
creating a kind of physical chain reaction
of oxytocin surging through our body,
lighting up cells with natural positivity.
This is the drug with the ability to cure depression,
whilst boosting our immune system to fight infection.
Uplifted by acts of genuine moral beauty,
minds kept sharp and our metabolism healthy.

Being kind. An antidote to conflict and stress.
Replacing heat of anger with thoughtful goodness.
Pass it on. Show gratitude when it matters.
A compassionate heart brings happiness to others.
Our self-esteem rises by making someone else feel valued.
So our kindness practices should be consciously imbued
with more love, more humanity, changing our brain chemistry
to strengthen our sense of purpose, thus combatting anxiety.
Plant seeds of kindness. Be a blessing. A ripple in a lake.
Communities impacted by choices that we make
to be kind. To influence society through simple psychology,
by becoming the people we want to be.
Better versions of ourselves creating strong bonds,
deeper friendships. Grumps, grudges, animosity long gone.
A positive attitude actually slows our bodies degradation,
strengthens hearts, protects cells from inflammation.
So increase your happy hormones. Get rid of resentment.
Kindness, experts say, is a natural antidepressant.
Compassionate acts are legal chemical highs.
Dopamine restores, reactivates. Let's be revitalised
to deepen our relationships with those we love,
or reach out to strangers. Sometimes, it's enough
to wave, smile, wish someone a wonderful day,
or help unexpectedly. Being kind is always the right way.
Even when faced with hostile negativity,
we can choose how to respond. It's easy spiritual alchemy.
Our children see our actions. Our behaviour speaks for itself.
A lasting legacy, not just for our own all-round health.
Each act matters far more than we think.
Compassion connects us. Through love we're linked.
Meditate, reflect on how we treat those around us.

Our world would change dramatically if we acted with more kindness.
So, if we want longevity, a healthy body, a healthy mind,
it's not rocket science, my friends, the solution is just... be kind.

CHAPTER 22
Let it out!

'Humour is the great thing, the saving thing after all. The minute it crops up, all our hardnesses yield, all our irritations, and resentments flit away, and a sunny spirit takes their place.'

~

Mark Twain

What can we do at the actual 'blast off' moment to alleviate tension? I spoke to a friend the other day. Usually mild mannered, she described how she'd spent the best part of her afternoon miming swear words out of her kitchen window! How many of us have been there? Locking ourselves in the bathroom mouthing obscenities at the wall? A perfectly acceptable defusing strategy, I would argue. Though I'd advise against facing the mirror though. Off-putting to watch ourselves mid mini-melt down. Witnessing one's own contorted face is most distracting, particularly at full velocity! If that's not your bag, how about interpretive dance? I've been known to indulge in my own unique performances of 'pissed off-ness' around the room. Not for public viewing, but very effective for the purpose it serves, also a good cardio workout! Win-win.

Whilst I advocate mime and free-form dance as a self-expressive outlet, there are less conspicuous, more measured approaches to emotional release – take writing for example. I cannot laud the benefits of expressive writing [31] enough. I've never been a consistent diary writer, but, when my stepmother / infertility double whammy arrived, writing about my feelings evolved into a great coping strategy. Marbles were frequently salvaged through a burst of writing! A cheap, easy way to get stuff off our chests, it doesn't require much. Just time, space, a pen and paper.

When busy and tired, and other life demands take precedence, prioritising mental downtime takes effort. Uninterrupted, mind-salving, personal space in which to re-organise thoughts, release pressure, articulate worries, or discharge frustrations is a helpful well-being practice. The more stressed and busier I am, the more I need it. When a week or two has gone by without it, I start to feel jittery. My writing takes different forms, dictating the seeds of an idea or poem into my phone while walking the dog, an early morning reflection, a late (or middle of the night even), indignant splurge. It all feels good!

Sometimes, I'd have still preferred to shove my head under my pillow. Or done a runner to the airport. But thanks to encouraging reminders from Vanessa, I kept jotting down thoughts and feelings when they materialised. In the midst of her grief, she'd found writing to be considerably useful. If it helped her, I resolved, then I too should prioritise it.

I could be quite distracted, practically tying myself to the chair on occasion. Nevertheless, I rarely finished a session feeling worse. Almost always better. Writing has cathartic, healing properties that serve to unburden a crowded, saturated mind. I asked Vanessa to share her thoughts on how writing had helped her through her grief.

'Writing helped me to process and confront things I couldn't talk about for one reason or another. Through writing, I began to appreciate the depth and magnitude of significant feelings and thoughts I'd assumed were insignificant. The very act of physically writing down thoughts facilitated many connections which resulted in shifts from what I describe

as mental blockages. Sometimes, you just don't need this stuff clogging up your brain. It once did, but now it's served its purpose, yet you're still carrying it. Writing was a way to clear out many of these thoughts. Writing doesn't change the facts, but it can change your mind-set. Useful when you're stuck with crap you can't change.' Vanessa

According to a 2013 American study [32], writing about strong emotions and feelings can relieve symptoms of depression. The study took forty people suffering with major depressive disorder (MDD) assigning them to two groups, those who expressively wrote for just 20 minutes a day for three consecutive days, and those who wrote about anything.

After just one day, the expressive writing group had significantly reduced depression scores than their control counterparts. Not only that, up to a month later the expressive writing group continued to have significantly lower, subclinical, depression scores. So, if you feel overwhelmed and haven't tried it, give it a go. Articulating and releasing one's thoughts on to the page is empoweringly liberating for a befuddled mind.

Initially, it might not feel natural, but trusting the process, letting go and seeing where it takes us, can begin to lift us out of stubborn mind-sets, allowing much needed shifts to take place. These simple, consistent strategies can be hugely beneficial in the context of infertility, trauma and bereavement. Quite recently, in fact, there's been an increase in written exposure therapy to treat PTSD which has proven effective in many cases.

There are many therapies that help us *'feel better, or grow stronger, especially after an illness'.* [33] Therapy can be doing something we enjoy either alone or with people we like spending time with. It can be simple, like writing. Or singing, meditation, baking, yoga, sewing or going for a walk. We need to factor it into our lives. What's your therapy? What do you look forward to? What balances out your stress and rejuvenates you? I asked Amy, my wonderful 'stars in a jar' friend, who had recently rediscovered a passion for painting, how it had helped her through her challenges.

'Art has helped me through an emotional and traumatic time due to the breakdown of my marriage. I loved drawing when I was young. I drew my ballet pointe shoe with ribbons. I remember how relaxing and therapeutic it was, and the feeling of achievement, doing something I was proud of. I never drew as an adult. Then one day, a friend of mine, a Cruse bereavement counsellor, suggested I write or draw my thoughts and emotions. So, tentatively, I got a piece of paper and started drawing – mountains, eyes, trees, flowers. I covered the paper with words too – feelings, aspirations. If you find it difficult to express yourself in other ways, using pictures, bright splashes of colour, scrawling words, and phrases that come to mind, might be easier.'

'My children inspired me. They're amazingly artistic. They rekindled my passion for art. A couple of weeks ago, we sat painting together on our canvases, totally engrossed for several hours. It was wonderful. Initially, I made excuses – not having time, or patience for it. Telling myself it would probably be rubbish anyway, so what's the point in wasting a canvas? I told myself that I'm too distracted, unable to focus on the detail needed for painting. Besides, I had more important stuff to do, like running around after the children, working, cooking, and cleaning – day-to-day stuff. I didn't allow myself downtime. I had tried meditation and reading, but I couldn't concentrate. Art has been far more successful.'

'I think Art therapy can help anyone who has lost themselves a bit. It's helped me find my inner-self again. It's a form of 'soul-retrieval', I suppose. Through any kind of trauma, we can lose our sense of 'self' and identity. Then we motor along in automatic, pushing emotions aside - taking the easy option, doing what we know best, getting through the day by keeping it all functional. Finding an hour, or even 10 minutes to do something we're really passionate about and enjoy makes the soul feel good again. Giving ourselves attention when we're grieving, like with infertility, or any traumatic, inner emotional turmoil, is a way to nurture ourselves, a way to heal.'

'Art therapy has given me space to reflect, a way to have downtime, well-being time. It's helped me find that bit of me that's been missing for a while - parts of my personality that I was disconnected from, the free-spirited part of the person that I knew was in me, but whom I'd lost after years of conforming to who I thought I should be. Good therapy should empower us to express our true selves freely, and as in my case, rediscover who we really are and aspire to be.' Amy

Creative self-expression is not everyone's cup of tea, but we all need ways to uninhibitedly express ourselves whether we've experienced trauma or not. However, healthy coping mechanisms are not only a question of output, but also input. Choosing wisely, where we can, who and what come into our lives, into our souls, being vigilant about it helps. Take TV or internet content for example. We have so much screen time nowadays. Often, we need to consciously choose what penetrates our homes, hearts and minds from external sources.

Neither my husband nor I are raucous laughter types, but we love to watch comedy together. When the whole infertility scenario first unravelled, it was a pleasure to come home from work knowing that the two of us would later be lounging on the sofa watching our *Flight of the Concords* DVDs that my husband had bought online (in the days before the monopoly of Netflix!). I loved the reassurance of the ritual of laughing at the same absurdly funny, non-threatening thing. It counterbalanced the more serious stuff going on. Laughing at something silly and mundane with him was relaxing!

A reliable, defiant sense of humour helps forge resilience. Finding the funny side, when there is one, powers us through our daily lives more intact than we would otherwise be. Much like Karen's earlier reflection about acting brave, the more we flex our humour 'muscle', the more we integrate it into our personalities, the more resilient we become. It's all part of that metamorphosis into replenished, improved versions of ourselves. As Oprah says, *'You become what you believe, not what you wish for or what you want. You become what you expect in your heart'*.

We can rise up using our various strategies. Although admittedly, seeing the funny side is often rather difficult. Even now. Infertility doesn't provide many moments of side-splitting hilarity, but the absurd pantomime that it can be, triggered my creativity and is how many of my poems took shape.

I've come to believe that humour is to our souls what sunlight and water are to life. Without humour, little by little everything else – resilience, relationships, self-belief, passion – shrivels up and withers away until just a barren landscape is left. We can't always get it right. Life is a journey, a learning process. I still have sense of humour failures, but I'm able to move on more quickly to a calmer, more objective mind-set.

Humour, resilience, courage, objectivity. All helpful when confronted by external influences like social media! Boy, oh boy, I've had to flex various survival strategy muscles with that one! Although, for me, its redeeming benefits do outweigh the draw backs. Social media's marvellous ability to defy distance, connecting us globally is a big plus. I continue using it, particularly since moving to Spain. Subsequently, it has kept me in touch with a host of vibrant and enriching people who would've otherwise drifted out of my life.

But, as with many things, too much exposure has a dark side. For those who are childless not by choice, scrolling through reams of happy family photos, babies and children can trigger an avalanche of unsolicited feelings. Some days the sheer quantity was torrential. But I'm not the Grinch stropping off into my cave at the sight of every baby on Facebook, and other people's apparent happiness! In any case, it has become the norm to share family moments online. And why not? If you're happy, own it!

Generally, I don't suffer strong emotional responses anymore with the exception of an incident at my grandmother's funeral. My father's side of the family is blessed with an abundance of children all of whom were present. The poignancy of the occasion wasn't lost. As one generation bowed out, a new generation of great-grandchildren had begun. A literal living legacy that was very much a focus of the funeral.

Both my maternal and paternal grandparents were family focused – proud of their 'legacies'. It's a source of personal sadness not to be part of this in the form of my own children. It's an area that still has the capacity to break my heart a little, especially when photos are taken, shared and commented on later on social media. 'Such beautiful babies we all make.' (*All?* Are you sure about that?) 'The next generation, I love it.' 'Our lovely family photos. What a legacy!'

Not consciously, but somewhere in that pesky solar plexus grief trove, I grieved our embryos, and what could have been had they survived. Family occasions would feel completely different for me. I'm not saying it's not joyful to be together, but the sense of loss that tinges these moments remains a burden. But where there is darkness, there is also light. My cousins, and my brother are blessed with beautiful, healthy children. I'm thankful that they've not had to experience our ongoing pain.

And I'm also thankful that I planned for that difficult in-so-many-ways day of my grandmother's funeral, by organising a wonderful letting go, recalibrating, reaffirming dinner out with a few of my closest friends the following evening. What a loud, laughter filled, liberating, spirit rebalancing, soul nourishing, wine fuelled gathering it was!

Social fucking media

qWuGP3N5H2

If I see another fucking photo of another baby scan,
I'm going to lose my fucking shit! I really fucking am!
Congratu-bloody-lations! You have a womb that fucking works!
Stop posting that shit on Facebook. For some of us it hurts.
Yes. I am bloody fed up. Yes. I will bloody swear.
For some of us unlucky sods, it is un-fucking-fair.

I bet your online echo chamber is full of shit like that,
hundreds of posts of happy crap from other happy twats.
Oh God, I wish I wasn't miserable. I wish I wasn't such a dick.
But every time I see these posts it makes me fucking sick!
I can't mute everybody. I can't unfollow everyone with kids.
But it would save my fucking sanity if I actually fucking did!
Another bloody birthday. Another baby shower.
Jesus! Unbelievable. I'm getting madder by the hour.
My feed's clogged up with photos. More twatting videos everyday.
Is there a button that I can click so the fuckers don't actually play?
More smiling fucking faces patting bastard baby bumps.
Oh halle-bloody-lullah! I'm in another fucking grump.
I don't want to see more pissing photos. Keep a lid on it.
The world doesn't need an update every fucking minute.
Oh, Holy Mary Mother of God, do we really have to know
every time your pissing child wears a novelty baby grow?
Your toddler's baked more cupcakes? How fan-fucking-tastic.
That photo's worth at least 50 likes. I bet you feel ecstatic!
It's not a competition. No need to convince us of your utopia.
Yes, your child is bloody beautiful. You didn't need to use a filter!
Happy fucking families. Yes, we do fucking get it.
You're super-duper really chuffed. I feel like total shit.
Oh, Happy bloody Mother's Day. Merry fucking Christmas!
As for shitting Halloween, don't be so fucking ridiculous.
Your child has carved a pumpkin. You've dressed your baby as an elf.
God, grant me the fucking serenity not to top my-fucking-self!

CHAPTER 23
Metaphysical fertility reflexology!

'Soul and body, I suggest, react sympathetically upon each other. A change in the state of the soul produces a change in the shape of the body, and conversely a change in the shape of the body produces a change in the state of the soul.'

~

Aristotle

Infertility, what a 'drag'! IVF, what a rollercoaster! Losing embryos, what a heartache! The journey is hard. We must find our support systems, factor in time and space to refuel and re-centre, respect our boundaries, and proactively support our minds, bodies and souls throughout the process. Especially if we're talking about years of process. Only once we understand, tweak and adapt our lifestyles to face our challenges will we be able to assert more control over our lives, reducing the feeling of being adrift without an anchor which causes much of our stress and anxiety.

Throughout the challenges, I found it difficult to just 'be' in the moment, in the present. I was often caught up with thinking about what had just been, or what was yet to come. Very rarely, did I put everything to one side to focus on being calm and still to give my poor old mind a rest. Many of us exist like this. Dwelling on what has upset or shaken us, absorbed by next thing on our to-do lists, or worrying about future uncertainties. Our minds never really disconnecting from fight or flight mode. In a semi-constant state of alert and anxiety, our bodies continuously churn out harmful chemicals and hormones that make us ill.

Now I've built in regular 'me' time. I practice regular meditation, yoga, walks through trees, or running along the river, or promenade. Moments when I don't think about life as such. Instead, focusing on my body and breathing, or appreciating my surroundings through sound, smell and sight.

The other day, a wave of stress had built up. An issue was really niggling me. But out walking with my dog, moving, deeply filling my lungs with oxygen, watching the bees busily buzzing from flower to flower, listening to the birds flitting from tree to tree, the negativity ebbed. Perspective gently began to uncloud my mind, even reminding me to laugh at one silly part of it. Though it's not always easy, the first plume of negative thoughts can be resolved and balanced by zooming in on little delights and wonders that light up our brains producing oxytocin, reducing stress, worry, and that harmful tricky customer, cortisol.

Back in the early days, I hadn't been so aware of all of this. Apart from the little hotel breaks that my husband painstakingly researched and booked, neither of us had a regular well-being practice. Reflexology with Liz was a turning point. In that year or so of nurturing mind, body and 'sole', more robust counter-stress and well-being habits took root. Although I had a fairly healthy lifestyle, I took more responsibility for my mental and reproductive health, my own all-round health, and continue to prioritise this.

Reflexology for fertility had been recommended by various sources, friends who'd supported their own IVF with reflexology. My consultant, and several books, also signposted both reflexology and acupuncture as complementary therapies, *'Reflexology is not a magic cure-all, and of course cannot guarantee a pregnancy, unblock fallopian tubes, treat chlamydia or cure endometriosis. However, by encouraging the body to work more efficiently, it can create a healthier environment for pregnancy to occur'.*[34]

So, though initially cynical, the idea that given the right attention my body could become a more foetus friendly vessel, was appealing. Before embarking on IVF, I'd hoped that my reproductive system could be enhanced. With unblocked, positive energy flowing more freely around my body, triggered by massaging the reflex points in my feet, perhaps, I thought, I might conceive naturally. Perhaps my womb might be able to lure a reluctant sperm into fertilising one of my dormant eggs.

Although studies confirm that patients can benefit physiologically and psychologically, reflexology still isn't a fully proven, endorsed medical science. Some are dismissive of its effectiveness, whilst others recommend it to supplement treatments and assist healing of various ailments. Due to my family's history, I knew that our nervous system is complex and powerful with still much to discover about its functions.

Take Phantom limb pain for example. PLP is a fascinatingly vexing phenomenon. My maternal grandmother, a quietly inspiring woman, had been a double amputee. In her latter years, both her legs had been removed below the knee as the brutal result of several debilitating illnesses. Though parts of her body were incapacitated, mentally my Grandma was razor sharp.

One afternoon, whilst trouncing me at Scrabble, suddenly wincing, she described the cramps and pains shooting down her lower legs into her feet. Staring at the empty space on her wheelchair foot plates where her feet should have been, I'd wondered how this was possible. Other times, she'd have an infuriating itch on her foot. Well, how you can scratch an itch if it's not there? Poor Grandma. She never moaned, nor complained about her disability. Sometimes, when on the brink of self-pity, I cast my mind back to all that she endured and am bolstered by her patience, fortitude and courage.

Like many amputees, despite having the original source of her pain removed, she still had significant discomfort there. In 2008, a study of PLP in ex-military personnel with combat related amputations found that as many as 50 to 85% of amputees reported pain in the amputated limb. This residual pain was characterised as stabbing, pins and needles, tingling and pressure among other sensations. The causes are still not completely understood. It's thought that perhaps the brain misinterprets information from the nerve endings giving the impression that the limb is still attached. The nervous system tricks the brain into experiencing sensations that aren't real.

So, though reflexology might be regarded by some as pseudoscience, I was more than willing to give it a go. As the relationship between nerves, the body's reflex points, and the rest of the body should not be dismissed. Did you know that we have over 70,000 plus nerve endings in our feet sending signals up and down our spine to our brain? It's not just the Chinese who've used hand and foot therapy for centuries. There's evidence that it was part of Egyptian and North American Indian cultures too. This ancient art of applying gentle pressure to reflex points to stimulate other areas of the body is said to heal and help all sorts of ailments and tensions, including infertility.

Massage is relaxing. Not much beats a good head, neck or shoulder massage. Unlikely though it may seem, especially if you're not a foot fan, having them rubbed and soothed can be equally gratifying. Lying under a blanket calmed by soothing music, candles and aromatherapy oils was the antithesis of stress. After a busy day racing about, seeing to the needs of others, ticking off mental check lists and multitasking to the nth degree, an hour of reflexology can offer us essential hit the 'pause' button time. Time for ourselves when we just stop.

I found Liz through the internet, and immediately warmed to her. The most striking thing was that she was kind. And right then, that is what I needed most, kindness. After the rejection at our doctor's surgery, and feeling so alone in my struggles, finding someone who made me feel valued, listened to, showed me kindness and was willing to take care of me on several levels, felt fantastic. She also understood my particular type of anguish, having experienced miscarriage and her own deep longing for a child.

When I first started, I'd be so wired after work and interested, that our sessions were possibly like interrogations for Liz. 'What part of my body does that connect with?' 'What's an adrenal gland?' 'Why is my foot so tender there?' I bombarded her. It's a wonder she could concentrate. Peering over her shoulder to the framed foot charts, I'd scrutinise what pressure point was what. Eventually, I relaxed and let go, slipping in and out of a kind of herbal narcosis as she pummelled. I slept so well those nights!

Be warned though. Feet are little maps of our body, gatekeepers of our physiological secrets! Eager to get started, I'd only cursorily filled in the basics on the preliminary health questionnaire. I'd not ticked the 'smoker' box as, I'd given up a few years earlier. Yet, this old habit was immediately unearthed. Working on the ball of my foot, the part corresponding to the lungs, Liz asked if I'd ever smoked. Busted! Her next discovery came courtesy of the tips of my toes. This time, I disclosed a recent sinus operation. Spooky!

And so it continued. How was my spine? Ah, yes. Slight scoliosis. What about my knee? An old sports injury. And my heart? The spongy bit in the left part of the ball of my foot was indeed painful when pressed. I confessed to a tiny heart defect. Extraordinary! But not the coup de théâtre. Gently pummelling my heel, Liz announced that I was ovulating. Was I mid-cycle? Weird, and entirely correct! Any lingering fears that I was in the hands of a master charlatan with fake internet certificates scattered across the walls were well and truly quashed.

There was also a display of framed metaphysical counselling credentials too. I didn't book any purely counselling sessions, (even though I was in need of them) private reflexology as well as private counselling was not an affordable combination for us. Mercifully, by the nature of her care, I always left our sessions mentally brighter – less tense, less overwhelmed, lighter in spirit, and more in-tune with my physical and spiritual needs.

Perhaps you're more informed than I was. My understanding of 'metaphysical' was limited. It had a mystical connotation for me. I half imagined Liz donning a starry, black cloak and pointy hat for when she counselled 'metaphysically'. Realising that I was an ignoramus, I looked it up. It was the great Greek philosopher Aristotle whose numerous books of thought and study led to this area of early psychology. A collection of fourteen books were posthumously brought together and entitled *Metaphysics* which is how it derives its name.

It was essentially a ground-breaking philosophy for its time, in 4th century BC. Science has taught us a great deal more since Aristotle, obviously. Many of his ideas have been superseded by scientifically proven theorem. However, it can be argued that metaphysics is the forefather of modern-day psychology. Many current practices have, at their root, the basics of metaphysics. So, whether you're a fan or not, it's hard to deny the influence of its main principles on 21st century Western thought, culture and religion.

Advance apologies to any metaphysicists if I botch this very narrow definition. My understanding of metaphysic's main principles is that it's the study of how we exist, existence itself essentially. What a whopper of a subject! There are many branches which combined make up this school of thought. One explores the relationship and functionality of mind, body, and spirit.

And over 2000 years later, we're still researching and discovering how these are all interlinked and connected. How one impacts the other. Mind and matter. How continual stress in the mind ages the body, weakens our immune system and even contributes to serious diseases and illnesses both mental and physical.

Metaphysics explores what causes us to be and what causes things to happen in our minds and bodies, and even how we impact others in the world around us, not just physically, but emotionally, spiritually and psychologically too. Again, it's the idea that everything, each of us, is profoundly connected. The ripple effect once gain. A reoccurring theme in my infertility journey. Another branch of my discovery!

I'll try it all!

A friend suggested acupuncture
with a specialist she'd seen.
So, there I was on my back,
serenaded by panpipes and a burbling stream.

A few deep breaths, teeny needles in place,
rebalancing vital energy,
this lady put her hands on my head
to heal me through the power of Reiki.

Warmth, relaxation, a sense of well-being
flooded through my body.
Minutes later I awoke with a snort,
maybe she'd unblocked my chi!

Another treatment bed, more soft hands,
this time my feet had all the attention.
This lady massaged, kneading tender spots,
attempting to improve my circulation.

Woozy on an essential oil high,
I could feel it dissolving my apprehension.
This blissful semiconscious state
was unravelling years of tension.

I floated out at the end of the session,
hopeful that my organs might soon react
to the pummelling and smell sensation
by producing hormones I'd previously lacked.

I started going to church again
where a kindly woman prayed for me.
Closing her eyes, lifting her hands,
'God,' she prayed, 'give her a miracle baby.'

My hope surged, as she whispered a verse,
Mark 11:24,
'... whatever you ask for in prayer,
believe ... , and it will be yours'.

Positive thinking, if I believed enough
maybe it would happen.
Perhaps this lady had powerful friends
and a direct line to heaven!

Books waxing lyrical about herbs
that boost female reproductive well-being
inspired me to see another woman
for some natural herbology healing.

Possibly the oldest form of medicine,
ingesting a combination of exotic plants.
This botanical practitioner described
how my health would be restored and enhanced

by prescribing a cabinet full of supplements:
vitamins, pills, creams and powdered variations.
This homeopath, mistress of herbal healing,
was queen of plant-based medications.

Each woman has shared her talents,
their skills soothed my stress.
Though it remains to be seen if the issue is solved,
my body has set the ultimate test.

But I've had a go. I've given it whirl.
The benefit of the doubt.
If it doesn't work, at the very least
it was worth seeing what all the fuss was about.

CHAPTER 24
Avoiding workplace 'emotional leakage'

'Woe-is-me is not an attractive narrative.'

~

Maureen Dowd

As established, I had little idea how the infertility circus would impact every area of life. No one tells you, and this is the nitty gritty that could really do with a heads-up. I needed a crash course. A TED Talk. An A-Z beginner's guide to staying sane at work would've been helpful. As per usual, I flailed around trying to figure it out. Making a right pig's ear of it! It's perfectly normal to underestimate how our work lives, and career will be besieged when long-term infertility becomes our Ringmaster. And if we're in the dark, then is it any wonder that many employers are unaware of how to best support their employees?

Slowly choking the fun out of our personal lives, infertility elbows its way into our professional ones too. If only someone had ushered me into a private cinematic viewing of, 'And this is the way it is.' The director's cut. A fly on the wall documentary of the whole darn thing, including when at work. In fact, in 2019, BBC Scotland's *Making Babies* documentary was a brilliant piece of journalism on the subject. BBC Radio 5 Live's interview in the same year, with three women having IVF while they were working is also insightful.

However, back in 2012/2013, knowing my rights and understanding how my employers could help would have made a positive, more supportive difference. Perhaps I would've established healthier work-life balance routines sooner, been kinder to myself, and had more realistic expectations at work. The guilt and shame I felt, (there's that word again!) that I was 'allowing' my personal life to seep into my professional space was persistent. When I felt like I was performing less than my best, it really battered my self-esteem. Unfortunately, my confidence, in a job that ordinarily I loved, took a pounding. The tight knot in my stomach at the effort of concealing how I really felt was draining and a nuisance. Again, I turned to friends to ask what it was like for them, combining work and infertility treatments.

'Infertility had a big impact on my working life. I worked in banking, as trader support. It was a very stressful environment with daily deadlines and long hours. I felt that this was too much to deal with when I was undergoing fertility treatment, as I struggled to have the mental capacity to work under that pressure for that many hours a day. At work, I was more emotional than normal, and although I managed to stay focused most of the time, it was a huge mental effort. I kept thinking that my work was not doing me any good. I felt drained of energy at the end of each week. I'd make it to Friday, then could not stop crying when I got home.' Dina

'I was self-employed, working with many women, babies or young children. I specialised in working with women during pregnancy and postnatally, so was constantly confronted with what I longed for and failed to achieve. It affected my self-esteem. It felt like I was failing at not being able to do what other women seemed to do so easily. Overall, I managed not to let it affect my focus when working, but it was always on my mind. It required a lot of mental strength to keep all the mental babble inside and not let it spill out to my clients. I didn't want to them thinking of me as a failure, so I tried not to discuss things. Although, when I was going through IVF and waiting for phone calls or results, then it was virtually impossible to focus on work.' Ruth

'Mental strength' is a common theme with infertility. Acknowledging the strength required whilst honestly sharing our experiences of how we've forged ahead courageously can be life-affirming, empowering, and reassuring. In order to feel connected and less alone, it can help to read blogs, interviews and personal accounts by women with similar workplace experiences. We can learn from each other, be reassured that we're not going mad, and aren't 'over-reacting' to the challenges of infertility, especially in the pressurised environments of our workplaces.

If I'm honest, I was scared by what was happening to me in my work environment. I thought I was cracking up! Even years after the most traumatic times, I feel relieved reading how it had impacted other women at work too. Self-reproach for not being consistently focused, feeling that I'd somehow failed at my job back then, still lingered. I've now let that go. I did my best under the circumstances.

Being able to speak non-fearfully to our bosses about how we're coping day-to-day in the workplace throughout the treatment process, would make a positive difference to many IVF-ers. Understanding employers is another branch of our vital support network. One that can quintessentially change the whole out-look of women in the workforce going through this type of thing.

Looking back at IVF No. 1, I was fortunate to have lovely colleagues, but sadly, in the absence of regular check-ins with an in-tune, on-my-wavelength line-manager, I was overcome with anxiety. Never in the classroom teaching, that always gave me a boost, but during meetings and all the other rigmarole. Combining treatment with work responsibilities was stressful. I didn't feel I could be honest about needing more support, even if it was just knowing that someone at work had my back.

Like Dina, my energy levels depleted rapidly, mainly through the effort of conjuring an upbeat attitude when I didn't feel like it. Exhaustion affected my concentration. And I couldn't interact normally with colleagues. However, the show must go on! We all have a work persona, but teaching... teaching is in a league of its own! In our profession, the mask goes on in the morning, we take it off on the evening. My drama degree came in handy much of the time.

I leant hugely on these skills. Especially in a classroom full of kids with varying attention spans, when I metamorphosed into someone else - my teaching alter ego! A classroom avatar. Cross the threshold, the curtain goes up, the follow-spot flicks on, and the show begins. Ta-dah! The one on whom all 32 pairs of eyes are trained. Entertainer, educator, counsellor, performer, even singer and dancer, literally sometimes.

Whilst in performance mode, we must simultaneously remain calmly confident, responsive, knowledgeable, patient and positive, and of course, operate the 'all-seeing eye'! When in full swing, troubles are categorically parked and compartmentalised! Even so, although never in front of the kids, having a wobble at work every now and then, through years of trying to conceive, was inevitable. Even for those who possess sturdy levels of emotional self-control, like Karen.

'I'm pretty good at compartmentalising, but infertility and my numerous treatments definitely had an impact at work. I made a conscious effort not to let it affect work, but definitely battled more to focus as my mind was constantly scanning my body for signs of miscarriage, pregnancy, or imminent period starting! But I'm a firm believer of stiff upper lip and just marched on.'

'The most difficult aspect of trying to be consistent in my professional role was emotional leakage! I try to remain as professional as possible, which

means I don't like having melt downs in front of colleagues. I think it's inevitable for everyone sometimes, but it's so much harder when dealing with such huge emotional challenges outside work.' Karen

Self-control at work was essential. No matter what pandemonium was going on behind the scenes, those plates still spun, albeit shakily at times. But, as Karen says, it's impossible to entirely separate professional and personal life. One day, soon after our first IVF fail, I couldn't contain it. The effort of hiding the grief became too much. But one can't succumb to 'emotional leakage' when about to preside over challenging, uncharitable, hormonal teenage boys! A sobbing, mascara dribbling wreck would've been an unmitigated disaster!

Springing into action one lunchtime, I slunk off to an empty classroom to have a good old private cry. Such an episode can be carried out efficiently with minimal fuss. It's when one has an audience that things get more complicated. This neat little stealth sob was over and done with in minutes. Once the overwhelming urge to cry is dealt with, one can re-emerge dignity and make-up intact, head held high, gathering one's remaining reserves to resume normal service in a stable, less emotionally volatile fashion!

I don't advocate this behaviour on a regular basis! But sometimes needs must. Preparation is essential for when it occurs. Keeping car keys (in case your vehicle is the only suitable retreat), tissues, mascara, lipstick, a small mirror, water (crying is so dehydrating!) and perfume close at hand is advisable.

Definitely perfume! A generous squirt could be the most essential part of your stealth sob kit if your hiding location happens to be a musty cleaner's cupboard. It'll mask any lingering whiffs of cleaning detergent, bleach or stinky damp mops! I never resorted to it, but knowing the cleaner's cupboard was usually left unlocked was most reassuring.

I should've reached out more to those I trusted and counted as friends at work. But again shame, and a sense of failure prevented me. I've said this often throughout; life teaches us such varying and tough lessons through retrospect and experience. Mine brings me back to many mantras. A few that have a work specific focus are 'Learn when to gently, but firmly say no.' (Just as Dina was suggesting.) 'Be truthful.' 'Find your support.' Also, 'surround yourself with positive, empathic people.'

Whether we're dealing with fertility issues or not, these factors are just as important in our places of work as they are in our homes and our relationships. What if we fear being truthful about our personal circumstances at work? Or what if we suddenly realise that positive, empathic people don't exist in our workplace? Then what the heck are we doing there?

I'm grateful that even when I've been unable to fully forge my own support networks at work, on the whole, my colleagues have been understanding and caring. I never faced outright negativity from employers or colleagues when it came to treatment. Sadly though, many women experience a distressing lack of understanding, and even traumatic clashes with employers regarding fertility and treatments.

If our work environment is consistently unsupportive or harming our mental or physical health, fertility speaking or otherwise, then it's time for change. If day in, day out, we don't feel supported, safe or understood by anyone with whom we work, then I strongly suggest that if we can, we start looking for alternative employment! When things aren't working for us, somehow we must address it. It's always best to be around people who strengthen our personal and professional confidence, rather than undermine or erode it.

Staffroom exile

Every time my back is turned
there's another pesky pic
stuck to the staffroom notice board.
It's a mean and dastardly trick.

I'm trying to forget about it.
Work is my safe oasis.
But even here I'm bombarded by
babies on a daily basis.

I've got a job to do.
One that I quite enjoy.
I'd rather not be distracted by
photos of yet another baby boy.

I log on to my computer
ready to tackle the day.
Checking my email inbox,
I find, much to my dismay

more baby birth announcements
with images attached.
Though I send congratulations,
I try to remain emotionally detached.

Later in the staffroom,
during morning break,
the conversation turns to children
as we devour homemade cake.

It's not that I'm resentful
of my lovely colleagues and their kids.
It's just I need mental switch off time
from my own failing pro-creation bid.

There isn't that much respite
from my frustrating battle.
So, it really would be rather nice
if work was free from baby tittle-tattle.

A pregnant colleague pats her bump,
another announces his wife's three months gone.
I try to keep my attention focused,
stay positive, in the zone, and strong.

Sometimes, I really worry that
I'm a terrible, bitter person.
But those that understand this challenge
tell me I'm like this for good reason.

Surrounded by incessant baby talk
it's hard to concentrate
on the job that I am here to do
without letting this baby talk infiltrate.

My mind's vital energy is being used up
trying to manage this additional stress.
I return home exhausted every night
from the emotions I suppress.

Perhaps tomorrow I'll find a quiet room
to eat my sandwiches on my own.
I can have a little breathing space,
essential recharging time... alone.

I don't want to be antisocial.
I'd prefer to have company,
but my emotions and my frazzled brain
require this sensible necessity.

It's not helpful to be on the verge of tears
at the drop of the proverbial hat
just because one is constantly
reminded of a cruel and cheerless fact.

I wish I could keep them separate,
work and this blasted infertility,
but it's not a strength that I possess.
So again it's lunch for one, for me.

CHAPTER 25
Career management

'Do in your heart what you feel is right – for you'll be criticized anyway.'

~

Eleanor Roosevelt

My first treatment was no secret. Some colleagues knew. But even when injecting hormones, stumbling about like an amnesic zombie, I didn't go on about it. I didn't want them to think badly of me. If I divulged too much about my tempestuous state of mind too, would that be held against me? I didn't know if it might affect my work records, or the attitude of senior management. I worried that mental health related concerns could be used against me later in my career. The fear was real.

I certainly didn't discuss anxiety. I feared they wouldn't understand – a top reason given in the 2016 Fertility Network UK survey for not telling an employer about treatment. Of the 28% of respondents who did not disclose to their employer, 80% did not do so because it's private, some fearing also that confidentiality may be breached. 50% feared that employers wouldn't understand, and perhaps wouldn't take their infertility seriously. Whilst 45% worried about negative career consequences.

On the medical absence forms, 'IVF appointment' sufficed. My bosses knew, but I didn't go into detail or officially disclose my first round. Meaning, no closed door, official meeting with HR or my line manager to discuss the fertility policy, or workplace protocol regarding treatment. There was no discussion with my employers about how treatment might impact me. I don't think most had a clue. I didn't myself until I was in the thick of it.

Had I spoken openly with my line manager, perhaps more guidance and reassurance would've been given; an overview of how to fairly balance treatment with work responsibilities. Maybe then the worries about what was thought of me, the embarrassment of 'not being my usual self' and fear about having a 'wobble' at work would've been quashed. Maybe.

It's not that I felt completely unsupported. Not once were my appointments questioned. And only once when not functioning at my best was I actively challenged - a dreadful conversation, very badly timed and mishandled by an inexperienced male member of management. Nevertheless, there were no actual discussions or 'acts' of emotional or practical support during that time from my employers. When I asked Dina about her experiences on this subject, it turns out that she too, had a rather negative run in with a male member of management.

'During my first year of IVF treatment, I didn't tell anyone at work. My doctor signed me off for the Two Week Wait. When I found out I wasn't pregnant, I was very upset. When I started my next IVF round, I told my bosses. The female manager was very understanding and agreed that I wasn't expected to work any overtime. My male line manager, however, would get very annoyed with me leaving after 8 hours work every day. I wondered if he had been informed of my situation, and the agreement about no additional hours.'

'There was one incident when he came running after me down the hallway as I was leaving. He confronted me in front of other colleagues, 'Where do you think you're going?' Oddly, it transpired that he was fully

aware of my situation. I think he lacked empathy and understanding about how treatment can impact a person. I ended up contacting HR for advice. After that, it was very awkward between us. A bit stressful, as subsequently, it felt like he was avoiding me.' Dina

When Dina first shared her experience, I had to suppress an exasperated eye-roll. How is it that a conscientious, hardworking team member can be treated in such an unempathic, unprofessional manner? As Dina and I both found, it's a gamble how much to disclose. We must do what we feel is right, appropriate, and what we can handle. Though, I'd err on the side of honesty, it doesn't always pay off.

In all the years my husband worked at a previous school, he'd never had a day off sick. When he requested to take me to hospital for the egg retrieval operation, despite his track record, he was refused, unless he took unpaid leave. His boss eventually capitulated, but only after it'd added further anxiety to an already stressful process! (Not the epitome of a supportive employer in several areas so it turned out!)

Attitudes and awareness do seem to be improving in the work domain. But, it remains rather hit and miss as to how well one is supported. I return to the Fertility Network UK survey as a benchmark. When it came to employers understanding the needs of employees having treatment, 59% of respondents felt that their employer would benefit from education and support to help them deal with the matter more appropriately and compassionately.

The practicalities of combining work and treatment is a minefield too. It's best not to book IVF when essential, non-avoidable commitments like travel far from home, key projects, or meetings are on the horizon. For the most organised of couples, IVF won't necessarily slide neatly into our tidy, pre-arranged schedules. IVF has to be THE thing. Top priority. There's a strict timetable, and even then, that can change in a flash, or rather, a 'flush'. A hot one. Every 'body' responds differently. If the clinic calls, telling you to come, you go.

Medications? Well, many need to be kept refrigerated. And must be administered at a specified time, several times daily, on the hour. Whilst the clinic and patients have worked out the treatment timetable, it often changes. Appointments cannot be dictated by employers, patients, or even by the clinic, but by what happens biologically. And no one, not even the most accredited assisted reproductive treatment technicians can predict exactly what will happen at each stage. Stress!

The female reproductive system primarily calls the shots, though clearly, the male anatomy has some say. Our amazing, yet temperamental bodies can serve up some extraordinary surprises, good and bad, at the best of times. During IVF, there must be wriggle room and flexibility. Many employers don't understand this because they're unaware of the rigours and demands of treatment.

No matter how perfectly timed the whole shebang is initially, in my experience and that of many others, it's unusual to stick to the schedule and avoid appointments during working hours, especially if your clinic happens to be some distance away. Having an understanding employer really helps!

My husband, a self-confessed workaholic, and I felt guilty about having time off, so were probably rather pedantic about minimising the intrusion into our work-life when putting together our IVF schedules. (I imagined our consultant mentally face-palming as we ruled out various 'no-go' zones.) Thank goodness for my faithful side-kick mother who accompanied me so often! What she doesn't know after our 4 rounds of ICSI, and my dear brother and his wife's two complex treatments, isn't worth knowing!

In fact, Mother would make a rather good embryologist. Great, calm bedside manner. Steady, egg-puncturing hands! Brilliantly soothing hypnotic voice that cuts through semi-hysterical, nervous wittering... Our final IVF, frustratingly, took seven months to gain 'lift off', due in part to busy schedules, but mainly to a humongous balls-up by the clinic and my own body's refusal to play ball. (Forgive the delightful, yet fitting, terminology!)

Fertility appointments should be treated like any other medical appointment. However, this isn't a legal obligation. Employers, like my husband's former boss, who require staff to take unpaid leave, or pressurise employees not to attend appointments are not breaking the law. But it is poor practice, and the employee may have grounds for a sex discrimination claim.

Trying to balance the demands of treatment with equally demanding employers is stressful. Taking time off can add to patients' distress. It makes a huge difference when an employer recognises that treatment is already emotionally and physically demanding, and stressful.

Employers should be mindful, flexible and understanding with adequate policies in place to protect patients from workplace discrimination, allowing employees sick leave in the event of failed treatment, which by the way, is their statutory right when signed off by a GP as too unwell emotionally, physically or both, to work.

If the daily management of combining treatment with work causes additional anxieties for some, then so too does the impact of infertility on one's career. It's virtually impossible not to consider our careers. I've wondered if notes were taken in a little black book somewhere, ready for scrutiny should I go for a promotion, or interview elsewhere. Would medical appointments be laid bare for potential future employers?

Thankfully, it hasn't prevented me from receiving promotions, or moving jobs. Others, however, aren't so fortunate. Swathes of women report missing out on promotions, and general lack of career progression due to loss of credibility at work. How infuriating! Being penalised not just in the short term, but longer term too.

On the other hand, some women, myself included, decide themselves to put their careers 'on-ice,' not applying for new jobs or promotions, relinquishing responsibility roles whilst involved in treatment and trying to get pregnant. I stepped down from one leadership position in an attempt to reduce workload and tiredness, focus on one thing at a time, and increase my chances of pregnancy. I knew I didn't have the mental energy, or strength needed to give my all to both. We decided to prioritise trying to conceive (which ended in an 8-year career progression hiatus whilst waiting in vain.) My career has 'suffered' due to these choices, and the challenges we faced. Interestingly, my friend Karen recounts similar career concerns.

'The impact on my career was definitely a worry. More from an absence point of view than anything. If I took time off would that be used against me, no matter what the reason? I also didn't pursue promotions because I was more focused on trying to fall pregnant and stay pregnant. I think one only has so much emotional reserve. And when something like infertility is taking up most of that then there is less left to use on furthering your career. Afterwards, once I'd accepted that this baby wasn't going to happen for me, then it was almost a relief to be able to focus on my career far more.' Karen

It's a shame that some of us feel we must make this choice. Sacrificing opportunities to advance one's career at the behest of trying to have a baby is frankly really rubbish. Choosing one over the other frustrated me. Men don't have to in the same way! But being sensible, understanding what one can realistically manage at a single given time, is wise.

For me, simultaneously managing both pressures, plus minimal downtime at weekends, and holidays due to my stepdaughter's visits, wasn't viable from a mental or physical perspective. But that's the way it goes for some... endlessly trying to produce a baby is an additional job on top of one's paid profession!

The impracticalities of trying to conceive

czX2uTNNDc

It's gone from the sublime to the ridiculous
this baby-making lark.
For us it's no longer fun rumpy pumpy
under a duvet in the dark.

It's a military operation
just to bonk when the time is right.
Been told to keep a diary,
so we do it on my most potent, fertile night.

So much for being spontaneous,
for not analysing what we do in bed.
Now I think about it all the time.
It's driving me nuts. I'm bonkers in the head!

I've even bought a thermometer.
It's my basal temperature I'm supposed to take.
Even before I sip my morning mug of tea,
now it's the first thing I do when I wake.

I note down all the details
in a daily fertility log.
It seems to me a lot of work,
but I've been told I must to have a sprog.

I've got to set the alarm even earlier.
It's like a second job,
writing down so many observation notes
in my journal thingamabob.

Last week, the planets had aligned.
My ovaries had sprung to life.
So I texted my dearest husband at work,
'Babe, come home. Time get fruity with your wife!'.

Needless to say, he was not impressed.
He had a deadline for a report.
'But, my ovulation stick's blue, we must have sex!'
was my exasperated retort.

Earlier, I'd locked myself
in the staff toilet to wee on that stupid stick.
But you have to wait five minutes
and at break-time you've got to be quick.

I can't have my already stressed-out colleagues
banging on the toilet door.
Whilst I'm sat there waiting,
trousers 'round ankles on the floor!

I shoved the darn thing in a plastic bag,
took it with me to go and teach.
Whilst the kids were settling noisily,
I rummaged for something out of reach.

I took the register under the desk
as I peered into the bag.
It's really not at all convenient
this ovulation charting drag.

But lo-and behold, there it was,
a visible thin blue line!
Straightaway I cancelled our evening plans,
so we could be in the sack before nine.

That evening I worked my socks off
to get all my marking done.
So we could get passionate and frisky,
be romantic and have some fun.

But as I approached the bedside
eager to do the deed,
my poor exhausted husband
exclaimed he'd rather 'cuddle, chat and read'.

'Ah, come on love. Let's give it a go.'
I urged him to find his drive.
But within five minutes, we were both asleep.
This is draining our conjugal lust for life.

The experts say, 'Don't drink! Don't smoke!'
'Try acupuncture, but don't get obsessed.'
'Remember not to get too tired.
Above all don't get stressed!'

'Keep the romance alive, get exercise.'
'Don't keep your mobile in your pocket!'
'Take a chemist's worth of supplements.'
'Follow a specific fertility diet.'

I've bought all the books.
I've got a library full of fabulous advice.
Trouble is, it's doin' my head in now.
A break from it would be nice.

I don't think the experts have ever tried
following their own helpful tips.
Because if they had, they would've found
that normal life gets eclipsed

by the stress of trying not to get stressed!
By the pressure of trying to fit it all in!
And as for cutting out alcohol,
at this rate I'll turn into a bottle of gin!

Trying to conceive is a continuous nightmare,
a gruelling, humiliating quest.
I long for the day when instead of ovulation sticks,
I can pee on a flipping home pregnancy test.

CHAPTER 26
Choice, change and courage

'You can't change the wind. But you can adjust the sails to reach your destination.'

~

Paolo Coelho

Finally, I'd had enough. I knew something had to change. I knew I would go completely barmy if it didn't. Choosing to change aspects of our lives so they're more in sync, more balanced, is a brave, self-compassionate act. Admitting and recognising the need for change can be daunting, taking a lot of courage. However, if we're living our lives bashing our heads against a metaphoric wall, then it must be done!

It doesn't have to be permanent. It could mean a temporary adjustment. Neither does it have to be huge. The smallest of decisions sometimes have the biggest impact. Quitting smoking. Or drinking. (Well, those are actually pretty big.) Deciding to care more for our bodies. To care for others more proactively. Choosing who we spend time with, how we communicate, how we use our words, and respond to others. We can kick some butt with the positive choices we make about our own lives, encouraging and empowering others in the process.

Courageously choosing to harmonise and reshape our lives, or simply making way for more 'space', also opens us up to new possibilities and opportunities. The struggle to have my own child alongside being a stepmother had sucked me into a state of depression which meant that change had to happen. For, if we don't act, sooner or later cracks begin to show. Then it's only a matter of time before something, our health, relationships, jobs, minds, (or all of it!) start to completely disintegrate.

Good change liberates us. It should give us more perspective to think and see more clearly again. Change also provides opportunity for reflection. When I've embraced good change to improve my quality of life, I'm happier which makes me a nicer person to be around. I have more energy and more of myself to share with others, and my relationships flourish.

A less hemmed in, less saturated mind, also leads to feeling freer, and more able to pursue more meaningful goals and aspirations, simply because we have the mental space for it. I was so encouraged by the fact that parts of Dina's story reflected my own that I asked her to put into words why she had chosen to significantly change aspects of her life.

'After a couple of years of not conceiving, I changed my contract to part-time, working three days a week. I hoped it would reduce my stress levels, and I was concerned about my mental health. Obviously, changing to part-time reduced my income, but the advantages outweighed the disadvantages. For me, the reduced workload helped me to see that I no longer wanted to continue in this work environment at all, leading to a complete change in profession.'

'I wished I'd done this earlier, but you don't know until you do it just how beneficial change will be. Sometimes, it takes time to realise that you no longer want to work in certain way or environment. So, after three IVF attempts, knowing I couldn't carry on in that role, I quit my job. I began studying full-time for a bachelor's degree in nutrition. Then, I pursued a new career, now I work as a teacher. I'm so pleased I made this decision. I don't regret this change which led to many good things, to what for me is a more meaningful profession, and to finally having the baby that I'd fought so hard for.' Dina

Choice is synonymous with change. Taking stock, holding oneself accountable for one's life, and, just as Dina did, choosing to adjust is part of a purposeful life! To get out of a rut, we must act when we have the chance. Sitting around passively, nothing could happen for years. Our lives flit past. Our frustrations grow, wearing us down. Before we know it, we're living in a land of 'if onlys' and regret.

If our hearts tell us to instigate good change and we ignore it, this won't lead to fruitful, contented outcomes for us. Of course, change is scary. It draws us out of our comfort zones where new, unseen challenges await. The 'Fear factor' can debilitate us. 'Better-the-devil-we-know' syndrome kicks in and we risk wasting our best years making do 'lumping' instead of 'liking' it.

We tend to talk ourselves out of a positive, but daunting plan, fixating on reasons not to instigate meaningful change rather than reasons to act. We're excellent at finding excuses. Fooling ourselves into believing them, so much so that they eventually paralyse us. We remain stuck in the same old unhealthy patterns and routines. *Like a new pair of shoes, change is good for you, even if it isn't immediately comfortable. You might think that if you stay where you are, then at least you won't run the risk of setting yourself up for a fail or to be judged by others. You know that things could be better, but what if you rock the boat and make everything worse? You know you're struggling to manage everything right now, but you haven't got the luxury to take a step back and figure it out.'* [35]

My work routine had become untenably lopsided. I'd noticed resentment building within me. Whilst my non-peripatetic colleagues enjoyed a less fraught day, I continued to lug my heavy bags between umpteen rooms, up and down stairs, and across town. I was fed up with the sting of windblown drizzle against my cheek as I waited for taxis that were invariably late. I was cheesed off with arriving stressed after the confounded bell, despite having just relived an episode of Challenge Anika, only to be greeted by colleagues tapping their wrists, moaning about my class noisily waiting in the corridor! Launching into a song and dance routine about French grammar before getting my breath back, unpacking, or being able to go for a wee was sending my adrenal glands, cortisol levels and palpitating heart into overdrive. It wasn't healthy.

I'd voiced my concerns to management, requesting part time of four days. Hardly revolutionary! I'd suck up the pay hit if that meant a healthier, more manageable balance. I could see how it was possible. My submitted proposal was awaiting a final response from the powers that be, had been waiting for six weeks in fact. I was still waiting when, out for dinner one evening with colleagues, my mother called me unexpectedly.

Usually, it was an emotionally wobbly me who called her at this hour. I scurried off to a quiet corner to speak. She was at my house having a meeting with my husband... about me. Apparently, they'd been sharing concerns. She gently, but firmly, informed me, that they had agreed I should leave my job. (Erm... pardon?) They didn't want to tell me how to live my life, but felt resolute. Clearly, I wasn't going to be offered part time. Perhaps my employers were just stalling to keep me in contract past the resignation deadline. And as the deadline for handing in notice was a few days away, I needed to get on with it immediately by telling my colleagues tonight that I'd be resigning.

This was crazy! Or was it? Mid IVF, the physical demands of my job were contributing to exhaustion, and I knew if pregnant would be an impossibility, particularly if I were to carry twins. We also all knew that should it fail, I'd potentially spiral to further depths and difficulties. I'd already begun to worry about both scenarios. Yet, quitting my job seemed extreme. We couldn't afford it. However, whilst my mouth protested, my gut was somersaulting. In a good way. Something within me yelled, 'Yes! Hallelujah! Do it!' And when our inner voice shrieks that loudly, surely we must listen.

My mother's arguments were typically measured and practical. Sums had been done. My husband had drawn up a 'financial projections' spreadsheet. We'd be alright until I found supply work. She reminded me that she'd made a career out of emergency supply work, and had never been unemployed. There are always absent teachers, she reassured me. A few weeks into every term, teachers start dropping like flies. I'd simply sign up with an agency until something part-time cropped up. A weight lifted from my shoulders, and a light flickered on in the recesses of my mind. Five minutes later, I broke the news to my stunned colleagues. Looking back, this was a pivotal moment, the catalyst for a brand-new chapter, and approach to life.

Not everyone can up-sticks and leave their job, but we can choose to make modifications once we've identified what needs tweaking and how to go about it. Some more easily than others admittedly. But it's possible. We have the capacity to bring about change.

We have the choice to change our perspectives too. A negative mind-set won't lead to a thriving, positive life. When we look for the negative, negativity and misery are surely what we will find. The same goes for positivity. When we're in dark, hopeless places, where all seems gloomy and difficult, there are ways to re-spark our inner light, and positivity.

As I've said, change often requires help from supportive individuals around us before we're able to see it. But once we've glimpsed it, and understood it, we can choose to move towards living it, even if the process takes time. In the words of inspirational holocaust survivor, Dr Edith Eva Eger, whose memoirs are quite remarkable, *'You can't change what happened, you can't change what you did or what was done to you, but can choose how you live now.'* [36]

And so, I was leaving my secure job without a job lined up. Risky. But right. At the customary end of year work bash, one by one various colleagues congratulated me for being a maverick, for being brave and for doing what I thought was right despite the risks. (I replied that I didn't feel particularly 'maverick-ish,' I was only doing what made sense.)

That evening, I had many surprising, memorable, candid conversations. One admired me for sticking to my principles, and rather than just talking or moaning, getting up and getting on with my goals, which they admired. Another wanted to step off the treadmill themselves to try something different, but felt too afraid of the risks.

Sticking our heads above the parapet, accepting the risk factor is essential to change. I'm not talking about being reckless or haphazard. I mean a thought through strategy where risks have been calculated. When doubt and fear creep in which is inevitable, for a small amount of rational fear keeps us vigilant, and stops complacency, we must call on those who assist us in carrying out our plans.

Change involves choosing to think positively. Choosing to be brave. Choosing to take action. Choosing not to be destabilised by those who criticise, judge, or compete with us (for we'll never please everyone. There will always be cynics and critics!) And choosing those who, instead of activating our insecurities, champion our desire for good change and support us through it without promoting their own agendas, or trying to manipulate our decisions.

For all of us experiencing setbacks, failures and heartaches, there comes a tipping point with the potential to redefine our lives, and lead us in new directions. Whilst the choices we make may not always dramatically change where we end up, our journeys there will certainly be impacted.

I realised that I didn't want to be the victim of infertility. I wanted to be the victor - to be in the driving seat of my life! I was no longer going to wait for something to happen, I needed to make it happen. Now, when I feel sad, I still strive to have a conquering spirit that as far as it is able, engages with life in wisdom, balance, kindness, integrity and purpose.

I still want healthy choices to be a habitual, ingrained life philosophy, even if that means stepping out of my comfort zone from time to time. Hence, I suppose, writing a book about something that still has the capacity to make me terribly sad, or moving to Spain, or repeatedly turning down full-time employment despite financial implications. I whole-heartedly agree with inspirational lady, Brené Brown whose books I've read and TED talks I've watched, when she declares, "*I want to be in the arena. I want to be brave with my life... We can choose courage, or we can choose comfort, but we can't have both. Not at the same time.*" [37] If you're unfamiliar with Brené's publications, check them out. I'm a big fan.

Embracing healthy, good change isn't a mind-set that happens overnight. Like most learning, it's part of a reflective process. One that takes significant effort, self-awareness, and loads of fluff ups. But, when I do stumble and fall, I'm more patient and compassionate with myself. Then it's a question of dusting myself off, pausing, and giving it another shot with the support of my closest friends, allies and family. We can all do it.

Choosing good change

DLu2b7qCP

'You won't find a part-time job in a good school locally,'
declared the acting head, taken aback. His tone, almost fatherly.
'Besides you're valued here with us, you're part of our community.
If I were you, I'd reconsider my decision quite carefully.'

'The students, they respect you. They'd miss you if you left.
And the team, it gels so well, the staff, they'd be bereft!
Don't take the risk. Is it worth the cost? Something you might regret.
Your hard work. Achievements. What about your career prospects?'

The envelope resolutely sat between us. The embodiment of my
unrest.
Months of careful deliberation, now on the table manifest.
I'd petitioned. I'd asked. I'd bargained. I'd done my level best
to problem solve, show them it could be done. It was a reasonable
request.

Part-time isn't a dirty word. It's not improper. Not a wacky, radical
notion.
It's not a slacker's ruse for doing less. Or for those who lack 'proper'
workplace devotion.

Employees who aren't full-time don't have iniquitous intentions.
People need balance. Part-time is healthy. It's one of many sensible
lifestyle options.

I'd explained a little of this philosophy. Not in depth, but the gist.
I'd described my work routine which was not a way to comfortably
exist.
Arriving late, out of breath, drenched. The lunchtimes that I missed.
Physically, I could not sustain a work-life such as this.

They'd told me to wait. They'd have a think, 'we'll get back to you
when we can'.
I'd waited for weeks with no response. Now matters were in my hands.
Whilst they'd umm'ed and ah'ed, or perhaps forgot, we'd hatched our
little plan
which I'd just calmly executed by handing my resignation to the
astonished man.

There comes a point where a line must be drawn. A final decision
made.
Yes. I risked unemployment, but even this wasn't enough to persuade
me from choosing a new path, from making change. No. I wasn't
afraid.
I knew I had to leave to feel fulfilled. I'd have lost the plot if I'd stayed.

What did change when I stepped away from all consuming slog?
I felt liberated, re-energised. We adopted a rescue dog!
We spent more time outdoors. On the beach. In the forest. By the
river. I had time to jog...
Six weeks later, out of the blue, I was offered a fabulous part-time job!

There will be those who though well-intentioned, prod our vulnerabilities.
Those who try to dissuade us from our attempts to reclaim priorities.
Taking a stand, breaking the chain, clears the way ready for other opportunities.
Courageously choosing good change invites infinite new possibilities.

CHAPTER 27
New horizons

'A visionary is someone who can look out into the future with great imagination... When you have vision, it means you're able to look outside your current circumstance and situation, able to see out into the future.'

~

Angela Manuel Davis

Well, I did it. I wrote the book that has been on my heart for years. My vision to encourage others who need it by attempting to connect through these pages is now a possibility. I haven't told it all up to present day, but this part of the story at least, is out there.

I wonder if I'll have got it out of my system, the desire to share and unearth the truth. Several close friends have said to me, independently from each other, 'This book is a little like your child. You have gestated and carried it, now you need to give birth to it!' The more I've written, indeed the more I've felt that. A cross between a beautiful, amazing, Beyoncé-esque miracle and an irascible, stomach bursting Sigourney Weaver-esque alien expulsion!

If I hadn't taken the risk leaving a job that completely exhausted me, it wouldn't have happened. One of the first things I did, was try. Of course, it's taken years to accomplish, but once I could see and think clearly again, my creative juices got stirred up, and I dared believe that if I stuck at it when I could, it was possible. The fact that sitting still for hours is not my natural habitat made it extra challenging, but it's done!

Not only that, when I felt very low at no pregnancy materialising month after month, I'd imagine a book in my hand instead of a baby in my arms. It was bittersweet, but something within my power to achieve and could actually make happen. Writing gave me the impetus to keep going, and a positive focus when I was sucked under by further trials and losses, and the darkness that engulfed me sometimes, particularly when faced with the challenging of stepmothering and missing my stepdaughter.

I think we all need to tap into our interests and talents, as I've said, be it focussing on crafting a gift, helping to raise money for charity, or simply encouraging a friend in need. Remembering to step out of our own concerns when we can, to offer compassion to others at a time when they need it, can lift us up too. I've learnt that the effect is mutually beneficial.

I was also determined that infertility would no longer completely drain my husband and I. Writing honestly, poetry in particular, as well as reading, and connecting with others has helped to keep toxic thoughts at bay. Expelling and expressing this story has given me an expansion of head-space, heart-space and confidence. I now know I have the mental resources and resilience to give more to others professionally and personally, rather than only just keeping myself afloat. In different ways, my husband and I both have the heart of encouragers. I love seeing him thrive too. Now, I have more capacity to encourage him in his desire to follow his path. Looking outward rather than inward is where we both want to be.

As for my unemployed status, I was looking forward to a leisurely sabbatical! I had a long list of things to attend to. But funnily enough, my mother's words held true. I never had to sign up with agencies or send off my CV. It's strange how things work out. (Or maybe, after all, not that strange.) That October, only a few weeks into the new academic year, I had a call from a Deputy Head I knew of a school in the New Forest not far from me. A school I'd had my eye on for a while.

Through the grapevine, he'd heard I was no longer at my previous school. He asked if I could come in the very next day to discuss an immediate start for teaching French and Spanish to cover a colleague's compassionate leave. It was temporary, and only part-time. He was apologetic, only three days a week. (Are you kidding? Music to my ears!) Apart from a brief maternity leave sojourn at a neighbouring school, I taught there happily for several years until we moved abroad. Quite remarkable really.

Had I not taken a leap of faith into the teaching wilderness, my dream job would've fallen into someone else's lap. I'd taken a chance that had made me available and the right opportunity had come along. Whilst infertility was the scourge of our lives, I give it credit for bringing me to a place where, had my back been turned, looking the other way, I wouldn't have seen open doors, let alone walked through them. Another of my life code mantras has sprung from this, 'Never sit with your back to the door.' (I mean that both metaphorically, and literally, especially in the school canteen!)

My husband and I don't have the perfect relationship, especially when we're both bone-achingly tired! No one does, for we're all perfectly imperfect! But, he is my best friend who has weathered each storm with me. Each time understanding better how to work as a team. How to listen to each other. We continue to learn about ourselves, and improve how we interact with, communicate with, and nurture one another. A stronger, deeper, more authentic relationship is a fruit of our challenges, and we love spending time together. It's a partnership that continues to evolve and grow just as we do as individuals. It's an adventure and a reassurance to continue to spur each other on. We have that to be thankful for too.

After the first IVF failed, that following September, before the new job offer materialised, instead of battening down the hatches for a new academic year, recommencing the annual cycle, I grew fitter and stronger. I started running again, or could be found marching round the meadow, along the sea front or through the forest with our new rescue dog, Faith. What a joyful addition to our family she was!

My husband unaccustomed to dogs and less enthusiastic than me about our new family member, was soon smitten. His smile when our dog goes bananas as he walks in from work, is wonderful. She's an instant tension easer for the whole family. It's well documented that dogs help reduce stress, and anxiety levels. She certainly works for us. She gave us a new focus for our attentions and energies, and another reason to have to spend more time outdoors - an essential part of our positive lifestyle reshuffle.

My very brief sabbatical also gave my body some recovery time to heal and rest properly. My mind took longer. It was almost a year before I was ready to go through IVF again. In the meantime, I began to reconstruct improved, more balanced versions of our working and personal lives, understanding the necessity of boundaries, trying to set a few more to simplify our lives. I wasn't sure how I'd achieve it consistently long-term, but as the Spanish say, 'poco a poco' - little by little / step by step. It was my intention to gently cultivate a more enjoyable life together, and with my stepdaughter, whether our baby arrived or not.

Aging still scares me, but I'm proud of the woman I've become over time. Without the aging process, it's impossible for us to benefit from wisdom through experience. Thank goodness I'm wiser now than I was say 10 or even 5 years ago! I care far less what others think. I've a better understanding of my own worth. And I'm far kinder to myself than I used to be. I'm also more confident when it comes to choosing or even filtering out who it's healthy to have in my immediate support network. Becoming shinier, happier versions of ourselves is an on-going process, but one we can learn to enjoy. We can embrace the evolution whole-heartedly!

Regarding never having a baby? I find it heartachingly tricky to accept that my body will soon no longer be pre-menopause, but maybe that'll bring a final sense of peace and closure because no matter how much I convince myself that I've accepted my circumstances after all this time, I still secretly hope. Perhaps it's a flame that needs to gracefully burn itself to the wick so I can fully move on.

I'm not expecting magical solutions to grief though. Grief never fully leaves us. It changes us, for the worse, or if we're courageous and honest, for the better. It quietly walks with us as we go about the rest of our lives. We can kindly accept this. But, don't have to be defined by it. If we set our intentions right, if we make it our purpose to live giving out light, like my little fairy lights in a jar gift, then we can rise and shine regardless. Also, we can encourage by reflecting the light of others back to them, to remind them of their own unique sparkle too.

Being a stepmother is still hard emotionally at times, but the joy my stepdaughter brings, even as a headstrong teenager, outweighs the tough bits. Every time she says she loves or misses me, my heart does a little flip. It's all worthwhile. Not every stepparent is in this position. I'm proud of the relationship the three of us have forged. I cherish our time together. I'm excited for the next phase of our lives as she continues to flourish and grow.

When infertility struck, the inconceivable happened. Coping with the transitions between motherhood, saying goodbye, and the cycle of grief, was difficult, and hard for many to understand. It destroyed my confidence, eroded my self-esteem, altered my personality, impacted my career, and nearly broke my marriage. And yet, despite it all, many positives have been able to take seed and grow.

I may not have my longed-for child, which makes me sad. I still feel that ache. But I now know that sadness doesn't have to be a permanent fixture. I embrace and am thankful for all the goodness that is in abundance around me. It's not always easy to be positive. Sometimes, I have a proper grump which is usually dispelled by either a hug, humour or kindness. (Thankfully, my grumps are far less traumatic and frequent for my husband than all those years ago!)

And of course, I still mess up my self-care, rest, balance, and compassion to others ethos because life is still busy, and I'm still learning! However, when my fuel gauge teeters on empty, I'm more aware of the warning signs, and how to top it up. This is in part due to fantastic, supportive friendships.

Often, my friends don't realise the impact they have on my well-being. Just by being themselves, they lift me up so I can forge ahead. They remind me that I am enough. They help me feel valued, and encouraged. It is fitting to bring it back full circle to the women, past and present, who make me laugh, who despite distance and their own concerns, empathise and care. These are wonderful warrior women who even when life is complicated for themselves, nourish the souls of others. I couldn't have done, and couldn't continue this journey without my husband, my family, or my friends.

Peloton of sisterhood

qeBWH5DDmb

Despite my flaws, I'm thankful for the woman I've become.
I know I'm far from perfect, yet I'm proud of how far I've come.
But I can't take all the credit, I didn't act alone,
I've been guided, loved, and reassured. I wasn't on my own.

The women who surround me, those I'm blessed to call my friends,
have each stepped in at different times to stop me going round the bend!
Even at a distance, when not physically by my side,
I sense their faithful encouragement, my fuel when I am tired.

And boy, have I grown weary of the trials I've had to face,
I've wanted to admit defeat, give up this stupid race.
But stationed all around me in strategically placed positions
is my peloton of sisterhood, my network of 'soul' physicians.

Their strength, courage, and wisdom is what's kept me in the saddle.
My resilience I owe to them, especially when my mind is addled!
Providing calm perspective when I'm head down in the mist,
whispering quietly in my ear, 'You can do it, girl! You got this!'.

My friends don't have it easy. These days who really does?
But it doesn't stop them giving patient, unyielding love.
Such empathy and warmth abound. Their friendship keeps me going.
A living energy that circulates, through my veins continues flowing.

Listening without judgment, true friends don't belittle what you say.
Their words cut through your darkest fears, helping light the way.
Friendship is powerful. Like food that nourishes the body,
the confidence it instils in us strengthens us on our journey.

Despite the layers and a brave face, a true friend knows us inside out.
No pretence or putting on a show. That's what friendship's all about.
Helping find lost marbles, recollecting past failures and glories.
Together setting the world to rights, sharing varied stories.

They're comedians, psychologists, life coaches, and kindred spirits,
talented extraordinary women, strong even when at their limits.
I'm thankful for their encouragement. Together we've guffawed,
rejoiced and cried!
So, I hope they're blessed, as they've blessed me. I hope they've a
peloton at their side.

May they be cherished and protected; they've so loyally supported
me.

When weary, I wish them refreshment as they strive to be the best that they can be.
Let their conversations keep on inspiring. Let them be vibrant, wise and kind.
These wonderful warrior women who even when out of sight, are never out of mind.

THANK YOUS

'In everyone's life, at some time, our inner fire goes out. It is then burst into flame by an encounter with another human being. We should all be thankful for those people who rekindle the inner spirit.'

~

Albert Schweitzer

This book exists due to the encouragement and interest shown by a host of extraordinary individuals whom I'm fortunate to have met over the years. Not once laughing or batting an eyelid at my naive proposal to write about infertility, I thank them for contributing by allowing me to delve into the most intimate aspects of their lives. Their candid accounts, some incredibly harrowing, have helped shape my own thoughts and perspective on this topic, ensuring that my observations reflect those of others, acting as a sort of rudder through this writing journey. I thank each of these courageous women.

Amy, thanks to the strength you've shown through your own adversities, your reminders about self-care and your enduring friendship, I know I 'can totally do this!' You're remarkable. Thank you. **Dina**, I'm thankful that we met that evening. The generosity with which you shared your story and experiences, so encouraged me. **Karen**, your journey had a profound impact on me. That someone could experience so much loss, and yet still be as grounded as you, is an inspiration! Thank you for trusting me with your story and for encouraging me. My sister-in-law, **Heidi**, thank you for generously sharing your reflections, and for coming into our lives at a time when we needed you most. We're so happy you are a part of our family. **Ruth**, it was a welcome outreach when you got in touch on a hunch. Thank you for your honesty and advice which helped sustain me through further tough times too. **Sally**, thank you for sharing your account as a mother of a woman enduring such loss and trauma, which is so valuable to this book. **Sarah**, many times I thought of giving up writing, then when I thought of what you've overcome, I told myself I could surely finish a piddly little book! Thank you for sharing your stepmother experiences whilst simultaneously and courageously managing your own heartache. **Vanessa**, I'm indebted to your encouragement. For being the embodiment of strength and dignity in the face of adversity, and for enlightening me with the importance of 'me' time without feeling guilty. Thank you for your consistent championing of me as a stepmother, and your valuable contributions to this book.

There are many others whose light, inspiration, advice, and friendship are deeply embedded in this book. **Allie**, you reminded me of the true meaning of grace and wisdom when I was at my lowest ebb. Thank you! **Delphine**, I didn't deserve such unfaltering belief that I could write a book. You never doubted, instead sharing your own deeply difficult infertility battles. 'You inspire me to be my best.' **Emma**, where would I be without your amazing friendship, and wise counsel to keep my mind sharp? Your insights never fail to keep a situation balanced. Thank you. **Heidi** and **Katharine**, thank you for your friendship that makes me feel so valued, for such a wonderful act of kindness; camping overnight on the airport floor because you refused to disappointment me! **Kerry** and **Lou**, thank you for your encouragement on the final stretch of this journey, galvanising me to get the book out there and reassuring me. Thank you too for bringing 'The parent plan' to life. **Liz,** thank you for caring for my weary spirit when I was on the brink! **Marie,** you were so candid about your own fertility troubles when you didn't have to be. It helped to open my eyes to the wider issue all those years ago. I'm so grateful. **Mat** and **Kat**, your steadfast friendship, vibrant positivity and creativity motivate and inspire me. Thank you. I want to express gratitude to **Sara Riseborough** and, in particular, **Shane Thuillier**. Your magnificent counselling and psychotherapy have benefitted my life in ways that can never be fully understood or expressed. A big thank you to all **colleagues** and **friends** over the years who in person or via other mediums encouraged my poetry and writing, for listening without prejudice, laughing in the right places, and saying flattering things!

I'm indebted to my family for their enduring love and support. My parents, **Gill** and **John,** for being endlessly encouraging of not only my desire to write a book, but also of my husband and I, in all our trials and tribulations. How did you become such understanding and accepting people? My parents-in-law, **Peter** and **Rachel**, your kind generosity was a light, and your home a sanctuary when we needed an escape. I thank my brother, **James,** for your love and admiration, and for believing in me. Also, my stepdaughter, **Emilie**, for making me a very proud stepmum.

To my friend and editor, **Emma Burgess**, for your endless patience, sparkle and encouragement. What fortune I had to be on that counselling course with you. Your insights, humour and empathy are magical!

And lastly, to my husband, **Jon**, thank you for rekindling my spirit on countless occasions. For being by side helping me try to be the best version of me. And for generally being a truly decent, kind, and inspirational human being. Je t'aime.

This book remembers Gloria, Vanessa's daughter, and William, Sarah's son, and is dedicated to all those suffering fertility related loss.

You are not alone.

'I've learnt that people will forget what you said, people will forget what you did, but people will never forget how you made them feel.'

~

Maya Angelou

End Notes

[1] World Health Organisation

[2] (Hodin, 2017)

[3] Assisted Fertility Treatment

[4] (Bolton, 2012)

[5] (Bradbury, 2018)

[6] Sarah Blaffer Hrdy, author of Mother and Others

[7] Sperm morphology is the size and shape of the sperm

[8] Human Fertilisation and Embryology Authority, 'the UK's independent regulator of fertility treatment and research using human embryos. A world-class expert organisation in the fertility sector https://www.hfea.gov.uk/

[9] Doodson, 2010, p. 123

[10] 2020's figures

[11] (Hamilton, 2008, p. 80)

[12] If you're interested in learning more, there are many articles, reports and blogs on the subject of IVF and mental health. I recommend a piece of great research carried out in 2017 by Cardiff University's, Sofia Gameiro and Amy Finnigan 'Adjustment to unmet parenthood goals: Systematic review of long-term adjustment after failed fertility treatment'. It makes compelling and insightful reading.

[13] Kjaer, as cited in Brix, 2014

[14] Kjaer, as cited by Huffpost, 2014

[15] Miguel de Cervantes, eminent Spanish writer of the 16th and 17th centuries

[16] (Chiu, et al., 1 March, 2018)

[17] (WHO (World Health Organisation), 2010)

[18] (Leanza, et al., 2015)

[19] (Sowislo, et al., 2013)

[20] (Venzin, 2018)

[21] Dr Maya Angelou

[22] Genesis 20:18; Hosea 9:11

[23] Deuteronomy 7:14

[24] Psalm 127:3

[25] (Voysey, 2013)

[26] Based on Dr. Kübler-Ross' model

[27] (Dykes, et al., 2014 p. 72)

[28] (Payne, et al., October 2016 p. 5)

[29] (Lux, 2019)

[30] (Hamilton, 2017 p. 30)

[31] Expressive writing is a technique whereby individuals engage in deep and meaningful writing about a traumatic or troubling event (Pennebaker and Beall, 1986)

[32] (Krpan, et al., 2013)

[33] Cambridge Dictionary

[34] (Dooley, 2007 p. 169)

[35] (Wasmund p. 58)

[36] (Eger, 2018 p. 272)

[37] (Brown, 2017 p. 4)

Bibliography

#FertilityAtWork, The impact of infertility on your career, and the challenges of combining fertility treatment and work [Online] / auth. Lindemann Katy // https://medium.com/. - 1 November 2018. - https://medium.com/@katylindemann/fertilityatwork-575b39eaca53.

'The desire to have a child never goes away': how the involuntarily childless are forming a new movement [Online] / auth. Marsh Stefanie // www.theguardian.com. - Monday, 2 October 2017. - https://www.theguardian.com/lifeandstyle/2017/oct/02/the-desire-to-have-a-child-never-goes-away-how-the-involuntarily-childless-are-forming-a-new-movement.

An everyday activity as a treatment for depression: The benefits of expressive writing for people diagnosed with major depressive disorder [Online] / auth. Krpan Katherine M [et al.] // www.ncbi.nlm.nih.gov. - 18 June 2013. - https://www.ncbi.nlm.nih.gov/pmc/articles/PMC3759583/.

Bulletin of the World Health Organization; Mother or nothing: the agony of infertility [Online] / auth. WHO (World Health Organisation) // www.who.int. - December 2010. - https://www.who.int/bulletin/volumes/88/12/10-011210/en/.

Childless couples have more divorces [Online] / auth. Brix Lise // sciencenordic.com. - Tuesday, 11 February 2014. - https://sciencenordic.com/childbirth-denmark-divorce/childless-couples-have-more-divorces/1396768.

Classroom behaviour [Book] / auth. Rogers Bill. - London : Paul Chapman Publishing, 2006.

Counselling Skills and Studies [Book] / auth. Dykes Fiona Ballantine, Kopp Barry and Postings Traci. - London : Sage, 2014.

Counselling Skills and Studies [Book] / auth. Dykes Fiona Ballantine, Kopp Barry and Postings Traci. - London : Sage, 2014.

Do less get more [Book] / auth. Wasmund Sháá. - London : Penguin Books, 2015.

Does low self-esteem predict depression and anxiety? A meta-analysis of longitudinal studies. [Report] / auth. Sowislo J F and Orth U. - USA : NCBI, 2013.

Episode 101 IVF versus PTSD [Online] / auth. Morgan Civilla // Childless not by choice [Podcast]. - 10 December 2018. - https://childlessnotbychoice.net/episode-101-ivf-versus-ptsd/.

Feelings of shame, depression and self-esteem mong women experiencing infertility [Report] / auth. Leanza V. [et al.]. - Catania, Italy : Obstetric and Gynaecologic Department, University of Catania, Italy, 2015.

Fertility Network UK Survey on the Impact of Fertility Problems [Report] / auth. Payne Nicky and van den Akker Olga. - London : Fertility Network UK and Middlesex University, London, October 2016.

Fertility Treatment Puts Women at Risk of Stress Disorder [Online] / auth. Rettner Rachael // Livescience.com. - 8 August 2012. - https://www.livescience.com/22194-fertility-treatment-ptsd.html.

Fertility Week 2019: #FertilityAtWork [Online] / auth. Lindemann Katy // https://uberbarrens.club/. - 19 October 2019. - https://uberbarrens.club/blog.

Fit For Fertlity; Overcoming infertility and preparing for pregnancy [Book] / auth. Dooley Michael. - London : Hodder Mobius, 2007.

Foster Mother-Infant Bonding: Associations Between Foster Mothers' Oxytocin Production, Electrophysiological Brain Activity, Feelings of Commitment, and Caregiving Quality [Journal] / auth. Bick Johanna [et al.] // Child Development, Volume 84, Issue 3, Society for Research in Child Development . - May/June 2013. - pp. 826-840.

Global prevalence of infertility, infecundity and childlessness [Online] / auth. WHO (World Health Organisation) // www.who.int. - https://www.who.int/reproductivehealth/topics/infertility/burden/en/.

Healthcare professionals not doing enough to address IVF trauma [Online] / auth. Walker Elizabeth // https://reprotechtruths.org/. - 24 September 2018. - https://reprotechtruths.org/ivf-trauma/.

House of Commons Library; Education: Historical statistics [Online] / auth. Bolton Paul // www.parliament.uk. - Wednesday 8th November 2012. - https://researchbriefings.parliament.uk/ResearchBriefing/Summary/SN 04252.

How to be a happy stepmum [Book] / auth. Doodson Dr Lisa. - London : Vermilion, 2010.

How your mind can heal your body [Book] / auth. Hamilton David R.. - London : Hay House, 2008.

If you forget everything remember this; Parenting in the primary years [Book] / auth. Hill Katharine. - Edinburgh : Muddy Pearl, 2015.

Is Low Self-Esteem Making You Vulnerable to Depression? [Online] / auth. Venzin Elizabeth // www.psychcentral.com. - 8 July 2018. - https://psychcentral.com/blog/is-low-self-esteem-making-you-vulnerable-to-depression/.

Is Maternal Instinct Only for Moms? Here's the Science. [Online] / auth. Gibbens Sarah // www.nationalgeographic.com. - 9 May 2018. - https://www.nationalgeographic.com/news/2018/05/mothers-day-2018-maternal-instinct-oxytocin-babies-science/.

Lisa Jardine: 'Nobody wants to run stories about the people who go through IVF for nothing.' [Online] / auth. O'Connor Steve // www.independent.co.uk. - Sunday, 3 November 2013. - https://www.independent.co.uk/life-style/health-and-families/features/lisa-jardine-nobody-wants-to-run-stories-about-the-people-who-go-through-ivf-for-nothing-8919813.html.

Men are from Mars, Women are from Venus (2nd edition) [Book] / auth. Gray John. - London : Harper Element, 2002 .

Message of WHO Director-General Dr Tedros at the 2019 IFFS World Congress in Shanghai, China [Video] [Online] / auth. WHO (World Health Organisation) // www.youtube.com. - 15 April 2019. - https://www.youtube.com/watch?time_continue=22&v=nTUN9MVE9p E.

Mortality in single fathers compared with single mothers and partnered parents: a population-based cohort study [Journal] / auth. Chiu Maria [et al.] // The Lancet Public Health, VOLUME 3, ISSUE 3. - 1 March, 2018. - pp. https://www.thelancet.com/journals/lanpub/article/PIIS2468-2667(18)30003-3/fulltext.

Mothers and others [Book] / auth. Blaffer Hrdy Sarah. - USA : Harvard University Press, 2011.

Oprah's Super soul Conversations podcast; Oprah and Dr. Gary Chapman: The Five Love Languages [Interview] / interv. Chapman Gary. - 20 November 2019.

Preserving snapshots of Cambridge's anti-women protests [Online] / auth. Bradbury Rosie // www.varsity.co.uk. - 13 August 2018. - https://www.varsity.co.uk/features/15985.

Rising Strong: How the Ability to Reset Transforms the Way We Live, Love, Parent, and Lead [Book] / auth. Brown Brené. - New York : Penguin Random House, 2017.

Social Relationships and Mortality Risk: A Meta-analytic Review [Online] / auth. Holt-Lunstad Julianne, Smith Timothy B. and Layton J. Bradley // US National Library of Medicine, PubMed. - 27 July 2010. - https://www.ncbi.nlm.nih.gov/pmc/articles/PMC2910600/.

'Still I Rise' - And still I rise / auth. Angelou Maya. - [s.l.] : Random House, 1978.

Study Reveals The Impact Failed Fertility Treatments Have On Relationships [Online] / auth. Huffpost // huffpost.com. - 4 February 2014. - https://www.huffpost.com/entry/infertility-divorce-study_n_4698074.

Taking charge of your fertility; the definitive guide to natural birth control, pregnancy achievement, and reproductive health [Book] / auth. Weschler Toni. - London : Vermilion, 2003.

Terry Waite: Faith Held Hostage [Online] / auth. Voysey Sheridan // www.hope103.2.com. - 24 April 2013. - https://hope1032.com.au/stories/open-house/2013/terry-waite-break-my-body-bend-my-mind-but-my-soul-is-not-yours-to-possess/.

The 5 Love Languages; the secret to love that lasts [Book] / auth. Chapman Gary. - Chicago : Northfield Publishing, 2015.

The Burden of Infertility: Global Prevalence and Women's Voices from Around the World [Online] / auth. Hodin Sarah // www.mhtf.org. - 18 January 2017. - https://www.mhtf.org/2017/01/18/the-burden-of-infertility-global-prevalence-and-womens-voices-from-around-the-world/.

The choice: A true story of hope [Book] / auth. Eger Dr Edith Eva. - UK : Penguin, 2018.

The courage to be a stepmom; finding your place without losing yourself [Book] / auth. Thoele Sue Patton. - San Francisco : Wildcat Canyon Press, 2003.

The effect of expressive writing intervention for infertile couples: a randomized controlled trial. [Journal] / auth. Frederiksen HJ [et al.] // PubMed Central (PMC), The National Center for Biotechnology Information (NCBI), United States National Library of Medicine (NLM), National Institutes of Health (NIH).. - 2017.

The Five Side Effects Of Kindness [Book] / auth. Hamilton David R.. - London : Hayhouse, 2017.

The really, really busy person's book on marriage [Book] / auth. Parsons Rob and Hill Katharine. - Edinburgh, Scotland : Muddy Pearl, 2016.

The relationship between stress and infertility [Journal] / auth. Rooney Kristin L. and Domar Alice D. // DIALOGUES IN CLINICAL NEUROSCIENCE. - March 2018 – Vol.20 – No. 1. - pp. 41-47.

Unresolved grief in women and men in Sweden three years after undergoing unsuccessful in vitro fertilization treatment [Journal] / auth. Volgsten Helena, Skoog Agneta, Svanberg and Olsson Pia // Acta Obstetricia et Gynecologica Scandinavica, . - 2010, September 17. - p. https://obgyn.onlinelibrary.wiley.com/doi/full/10.3109/00016349.2010.512063.

Women do better when they have a group of strong female friends, study finds [Online] / auth. Lux Helen // Upworthy. - 03 December 2019. - https://www.upworthy.com/women-female-friends-more-successful.

World Fertility Report 2015 [Report] / auth. UN (United Nations). - https://www.un.org/en/development/desa/population/publications/pdf/fertility/wfr2015/worldFertilityReport2015.pdf : United Nations, December, 2017.

Zita West's Guide to getting pregnant [Book] / auth. West Zita. - London : Harper Thorsons, 2005.

Printed in Great Britain
by Amazon